The
Trust Your True Nature
Low-Carb Lifestyle

Unleash Your Inner Carnivore and
Restore Your Health

Tracy A. Matesz

The Trust Your True Nature Low-Carb Lifestyle

Unleash Your Inner Carnivore and Restore Your Health

by Tracy A. Matesz, CCHt, Holistic Health Coach, MA Oriental Medicine (MAOM)

**Integrity Press
2018**

Please note that this is intended as educational in nature, and not as a substitute for the advice of your physician. We suggest seeking out physicians who keep abreast of the most current research. As always, your health is your responsibility. Mind it well!

The Trust Your True Nature Low-Carb Lifestyle

First Edition

COPYRIGHT © 2018
TRACY A. MATESZ

ISBN-13: 978-1981400812

ISBN-10: 1981400818

Preface

The original title for this book was *The Trust Your True Nature (TYTN) Low-Carb Diet Plan*. Centuries ago, the term *diet* (or from Greek, *diata*), simply meant *a prescribed way of life*.

Thanks to a suggestion from a friend reminding me that many perceive the word *diet* as a temporary restriction of food in order to lose weight, I changed the title to *The Trust Your True Nature Low-Carb* **Lifestyle**.

While we all want quick results, the body has its own pace and physiological limitations. What you eat should be one factor of many that define your *way of life*. The goal being to create harmonious and enjoyable practices that can be sustained long-term, and that nurture your physical, mental, emotional, and even spiritual well-being.

We believe that this lifestyle can help you best realize your full physical potential, creating the conditions to live a more purpose-filled life. We know that once you learn to *trust your true nature*, the rest is inevitable.

CONTENTS

1 INTRODUCTION

My first book, *Make Every Bite Count, Elevate Your Choices, Lose Weight & Feel Great ~ The SASSY ~ Super Affordable, Simple, Satisfying & Yummy ~ Produce-Rich, Plant-Based Way to Health (MEBC)* featured information and recipes that supported a whole-foods, plant-based alternative to what I considered the 'typical Western diet.'

As I wrote in that, and subsequent books, I adopted a whole-foods, produce-rich, low-fat vegan diet to heal an advanced case of fibrocystic breast tenderness, with noticeably fatty, enlarged, and uneven-sized breasts that were excruciatingly tender. I also had a myriad of typical health complaints ~ low-blood sugar, constipation and other digestive issues, allergies and ongoing phlegm and congestion, just to name a few.

Don had several of his own health concerns, including psoriasis, and symptoms of prostatitis for which he has a family history of both prostate and skin cancers.

We had immediate relief of our most troubling, potentially pre-cancerous symptoms within just a few months of eating our produce-rich vegan diet.

We subsequently immersed ourselves in all the literature and scientific studies we could find, much of which was written by various doctors turned low-fat, plant-based diet advocates. I was so sold from the swift recovery, that I completed the certification program in Plant-Based Nutrition, created by T. Colin Campbell ~ author of *The China Study*, and *Whole* ~ and offered through e-Cornell. I subsequently completed another online course to become a macrobiotic counselor and published three more books about macrobiotic diets following *MEBC* ~ all now removed from print.

In T. Colin Campbell's class, we learned that there are three main stages to cancer development. The initiation stage, where the conditions are right for either an endogenous pathogen, or for one's own genetic propensity to have cancer is initiated. The second stage is the longest stage, where cells divide and multiply. This was called the cancer, or tumor promotion stage, where a tiny cancerous cell can take ten years to become big enough to actually palpate, or detect through medical imagery, such as a breast exam.

This stage was considered the crucial stage, for as Campbell *claimed to have* discovered during his decades-long research, tumors could "be turned on or off" depending on one's diet. According to Campbell, rats that were injected with aflatoxin, a known carcinogen, would have rapid tumor growth when given *isolated* animal protein, in the form of casein milk protein, while the tumors would shrink when given a plant-based protein derived from wheat. However, I later better understood how concentrated amounts of an isolated nutrient is not recognized by the body in the same way as the whole food, something Campbell himself writes about in his second book, *Whole*.

At the time, we became convinced that a whole-foods, plant-based diet offered protection from many modern diseases, as put forward by his research and the work of other doctors, such as Dr. Neal Barnard, Dr. John McDougall, and Dr. Caldwell Esselstyn Jr.

Just prior to our making the transition, Don's first wife announced she had breast cancer. They had together eaten a Paleo diet, higher in animal protein ~ yet still containing moderate amounts of carbohydrates ~ for ten years, the length of time it takes for a cancer cell to become detectable.

Given Don's family history, and our own potentially pre-cancerous symptoms, we transitioned away from the animal-centered Paleo diet we were consuming, to a produce-rich, plant-based diet, believing it was the *animal foods and fats* that were the culprits of our health issues, as many seemed to be advocating. In actuality, prior to the Industrial Revolution, animal foods *were the healthy principal staples* of the Western diet.

While we did have a swift recovery of our more troubling symptoms, other symptoms never healed like we expected. In macro-biotic teachings, it is believed that since it takes seven years for the cells of the entire body to totally regenerate, some deeper/older or more chronic issues can take up to seven years or longer to resolve. So, we patiently waited, all the while continuing to eat daily bunches of kale, bok choy, collards, or other dark leafy greens, sea vegetables, beans, lentils, tofu, a variety of whole cooked grains, and small amounts of nuts, seeds, and fruit.

A 'nutrient-dense' diet, right?

About three years in, I began to have an increasingly difficult time getting going in the morning. I had puffy, tired looking eyes on a regular basis. It took me a while to feel ready for the day.

I also wasn't sleeping very well, especially during allergy season. I had been allergic to ragweed and pollen since age four, but my hay fever allergy symptoms were primarily in the fall. In the Phoenix, Arizona area, something is in bloom year round. I have been especially allergic to the wonderful broad-leafed shade trees right outside our balcony and bedroom window. You can actually watch these trees send out smoke signals of pollen.

A new pattern emerged. Each winter, for *five* winters in a row, I got fairly sick. In late 2012, during our high-raw, fruit-based experiment, I even had what looked similar to an adult case of Chicken Pox (despite having as a kid), with major chills and fever. About the time I would recover from the winter bug, allergy season would kick in.

I was dealing with ongoing phlegm, congestion, and a non-stop runny nose for several months. In early 2017, I completely lost my voice. Previous to this, I had never lost my voice to the extent I did, *ever*. I was actually scared I damaged my vocal cords. My eyes were also often quite irritated, red, and/or very itchy. Essentially, I began the first three months of each year feeling like crap.

Meanwhile, I was immersed in the online macrobiotic training, and an intense in-person and separate online yoga teacher training programs, along with writing books, and co-managing our clinic. Did I mention that I was also cooking most of our fairly labor-intensive meals of 'grains, greens, and beans' ~ the catch-phrase I used in my books?

Don and I started to see a chiropractor, as he had re-triggered old injuries to his back and knee that were not recovering well. I was taking yoga to help me with my own aches, as I felt continually out of whack physically, also a result of postural misalignment and previous injuries and occupational demands.

As my weariness deepened, I watched as new lines 'suddenly appeared' on my face at a too frequent pace. My frustration was growing too. I also had on and off constipation, despite my high-fiber, entirely vegan diet.

The chiropractor gave me my wake up call. He essentially said I appeared to be a poster child for 'adrenal fatigue.' Yes, I concurred. But I rationalized that it was the intensity of the yoga program, and did my best to hang in there and finish. I was not yet ready to consider that my so-called 'healthy' diet was not providing me with what I needed. But that is how self-denial and self-deception work. We delude ourselves into believing *everything is fine* to avoid facing the truth.

What happened to all those anti-oxidant rich plant foods I was eating? My fatigue, dry and ashen skin tone, and dulling hair reflected my weakening system, which was becoming ever more obvious to others, as I later discovered.

I also felt an increasing desire for more and more protein. We were eating up to 2 cups of beans, and tofu or tempeh nearly every day, along with the whole grains, dark leafy greens, nuts and seeds. Many plant-based diet followers ~ or dare I say fanatics ~ believed we were eating *too much* protein. Meanwhile, Don and I continually felt like we couldn't get enough.

We began to consume more pre-made, plant-based 'meats.' These were more savory, and somewhat more satisfying, but their novelty also quickly wore off. We were becoming less and less satisfied, and sated by our plant-based meals.

As I wrote on the Trust Your True Nature ~ also called Strong Spirit Woman ~ website, one day, Don had an epiphany. His epiphany became the inspiration behind the website and *The Trust Your True Nature Low-Carb Diet Plan/Lifestyle.*

Essentially, Don thought, "What if we were to choose from among those foods found abundantly in Nature ~ provided by God, or The Creator ~ that could be procured and consumed with a minimal level of technology (and possibly a heat source). What would we choose to eat?"

Man, and especially those of European descent from colder climates were hunter-gatherers (HGs) for the bulk of existence. We have historically consumed animal flesh foods, fish, and sea foods as primary staples, only to be *supplemented* by various assorted seasonally and locally available plant foods, including smaller, and much less sweet wild fruits, some nuts, greens and other above ground vegetables, and underground tubers.

At some point, early man learned to preserve foods by drying, curing, and smoking long before refrigeration and other technology existed. These foods were all provided by Nature, not a factory.

The advent of grains and beans is much more recent, evolutionarily speaking, arising with the Agricultural Revolution some ten thousand years ago. By contrast, our early ancestors, dating back to the Stone Ages and Neanderthal Man, were eating what they could forage, fish, or hunt *seasonally*, and *within their particular region* ~ two very 'macrobiotic' concepts that we do our best to adhere to today.

After Don's epiphany, we again transitioned back to eating an animal-centered diet. We now understand that an excess of *all* carbohydrates ~ especially refined, and sugary high-glycemic foods, such as bread and cookies, *but also* grains, potatoes and other starches ~ likely contribute to our nation's escalating rates of obesity, diabetes, and heart disease. Saturated fats and red meat require far less insulin production than carbohydrates, so do not promote these diseases. (Refined vegetable oils also play a role, as discussed Chapter 5.)

As a petite woman, past menopause, I have to be especially diligent with my diet. If I over eat, it shows quickly. To most observers, I never looked fat. But up close, underneath my garments, I had clear fat accumulation, especially in my lower abdomen, buttocks, and thighs. I have long joked about my lower belly 'kangaroo pouch' that never went away while eating a high-carbohydrate diet.

After Don's epiphany, we realized just how many ways that we ~ individually and collectively ~ have lived counter to our true nature.

For starters, isn't it interesting that *no other animal seems confused about what to eat?* We are part of Nature, yet we live as if we are entirely separate. And we continually give our power away to 'experts' while negating our own direct experiences.

We accept as gospel various ideologies, such as "saturated fat and red meat are bad for you" without examining whether studies validate the claim. As Dr. Wolfgang Lutz, M.D., and Christian B. Allan, Ph.D., authors of *Life Without Bread, How A Low-Carbohydrate Diet Can Save Your Life* point out, saturated fats *were never actually proven to cause heart disease*. In fact, there is no known toxicity levels for saturated fats, yet there is a *clear level of toxicity from overconsumption of carbohydrates*. Once upon a time, the standard treatment plan for type 2 diabetics *was* a low-carb diet.

Don's epiphany led us to question, if we were to set aside **all** ideologies, moral arguments and preconceived notions about what is healthy ~ *what would we be most drawn to consuming* if given the choice of those foods available *directly from Nature*, that could be prepared with minimal technology?

What if *you* were to choose those foods *you* are ***most innately drawn to eating*** ~ aside from what you *believe* you should or should not eat for whatever reason ~ choosing from among all those foods directly available from nature with minimal processing ~ animal foods and fats including meats, fish, seafoods, and dairy; fruits, greens and vegetables, tubers, nuts, and seeds ~ what would *you* choose to eat?

You may already be gleefully imagining your preferred choices in your mind, conjuring up images of a nice juicy steak, followed by some berries with *real* freshly whipped heavy cream or sour cream.

Then again, you may have an inner voice telling you that "Those are just *guilty pleasures*, and even if I *did* want that steak, it certainly *couldn't* be good for me." We have heard clients say, "I *can't* eat meat because I can't digest it." Or, "Meat makes me constipated."

Can we overcome our entrenched belief systems, and learn to eat more intuitively? Can we realize better health by learning to *trust our true nature?*

I believe we can, but we must first be clear about which foods are *not* among those found in nature, and available with minimal technology, and that could be edible raw if needed. These are foods you will want to avoid or greatly minimize in your diet.

Don and I are now pretty convinced that *we are indeed* more physiologically adapted to eating a diet that is similar to our Neanderthal and Paleolithic ancestors. We still have very similar DNA. It takes thousands of years before genetic mutations begin to manifest ~ much longer than since the onset of agricultural foods.

While several of the plant-based diet advocates believe we must fight *against* our natural cravings ~ *as if our human physiology is innately flawed* ~ we believe that if you begin to *trust your true nature,* you will be guided to make the best choices *for you.* It's really only your *mind* that gets in the way of your following your own *natural* instincts.

You *can* learn to tune into what your *body* is craving and discern among what may seem like mixed messages. You may have to unravel some long-held, erroneous and/or misinformed beliefs in order to start making choices that better support your ability to realize your present and future health goals.

Don and I have now experimented with pretty much every major dietary formulation from low-fat, high-carb to high-fat, low-carb, and everything in between, including eating a wheat and gluten-free paleo diet, and a high-raw, fruit-based diet. Our primary staple foods ranged from raw fruits and vegetables, to whole grains, beans and vegetables, then to animal proteins and fats with varying amounts of plant foods.

We have read research presented from advocates and doctors on both sides of the dietary spectrum. It is easy to understand how confusing it can be to the general public when there is such seemingly conflicting 'evidence' ~ often the same study being cited by both sides as validation for their *mutually contradictory* theories!

Suffice it to say, human health began to decline after the advent of the Agricultural Revolution. Populations world-wide exhibited diminished stature, and increased dental decay and nutritional deficiencies.[1] Ancient Egyptians who consumed a high-carbohydrate diet, with stone-ground bread as a staple food suffered from obesity, diabetes, and dental decay,[2] whereas populations eating traditional animal-based diets such as the Inuit Eskimos maintained better physical

---

[1] *Stature and Robusticity During the Agricultural Transition: Evidence from the Bioarchaeological Record,* Science Direct, https://www.sciencedirect.com/science/article/pii/S1570677X11000402

[2] *Obesity in Ancient Egypt* - The blog of Michael Eades, M.D. https://proteinpower.com/drmike/2007/07/01/obesity-in-ancient-egypt/

health, with minimal to no dental deterioration.[3]

We now no longer choose foods according to what we once *thought* or *believed* to be best, and instead make choices according to what we have *experientially* found to actually be helping us to realize our health goals.

In lieu of filling these pages with lots of scientific explanation, I have listed a few books and resources that I have personally found very helpful.

I do not make any promises about effortless weight loss or miraculous health recoveries, nor have I created dietary plans with a precise ratio of macronutrients for you to consume. Instead, I encourage you to follow your own inner cues, and learn *to trust your own true nature*, which I believe is far more empowering.

Getting healthy is an art. Each individual will need to find their own path. It depends in part on your genetic predisposition. But there is

---

[3] *Nutrition and Physical Degeneration*, Weston A. Price, D.D.S.

much more to it then following the standard advice of the day. In fact, sometimes it may require making a lot of mistakes first in order to really dial in what your particular mind, body and soul require for healing.

It is a process that will differ for each of us depending on how long we've been enduring unhealthful habits, how chronic our current condition, and how attached we are to our long-held beliefs about what is 'right.'

Probably more than any other factor, our ability to heal depends on our minds. Any ways in which we are living *against our true nature* will be reflected in our symptoms ~ whether physical, mental or emotional. If we are operating against ourselves, how can we possibly expect to be 'whole'?

The more in denial, self-deceptive, and/or attached we are to outmoded belief systems, or the more we engage in certain ~ often unhealthful ~ behaviors as a form of escape, the more challenging will be the healing process. You simply will experience what you experience until you are ready to experience something else. Often, the most intelligent among us are the toughest nuts to crack.

Healing may require some really challenging *inner* work. It takes courage to go against the tide. It is human nature to fear ridicule and rejection. To heal we must learn to trust ourselves, yet not believe everything we *think*, and everything 'the experts' think.

There simply are *no magic bullets*. The sooner people give up looking for the quick fix, and stop giving their power away to external sources, the *more elegant* will be the journey to a healed state. A state where you can become mindful of a symptom, and know how to self-correct, honoring your body's own well-regulated process of continually striving to achieve homeostasis.

Your symptoms become your cues to make adjustments. You are your own best teacher, but you simultaneously need to be the diligent and mindful student, paying attention to what life is trying to show you is out of balance through your symptoms, struggles, and sources of discontent.

We believe this guide can help you get on the right track, but, you have to do the work. Some people claim they want to improve their health, yet they are not willing to consider that what they *believe* to be healthy may not be healthy *for them*. Plus, the desire and motivation to make positive changes must be stronger than the challenge of over coming our inertia, and resistance to change. Our built-in homeostatic mechanisms also send off 'alarms' when we make too drastic changes too quickly, snapping us back to our previous 'set-points.'

It can be difficult to realize that our long cherished beliefs may actually be wrong, or to face certain aspects of our lives that we really *don't want to face*. Hence we keep ourselves very busy, and/or engage in various behaviors to remain distracted.

Animals, including humans, are wired to avoid pain and discomfort. Yet when we face our discomforts, we are rewarded with the greatest opportunities to actually heal our lives.

Following is what you will find in *The TYTN Low-Carb Lifestyle/Diet Plan*: Chapter 2 includes a list of the primary staples to be *enjoyed freely.* Chapter 3 lists supplementary foods that one must approach *with caution* as per one's tolerance. Chapter 4 includes foods that one should *minimize.* Chapter 5 includes those foods that everyone should *exclude*, most of the time, because they have harmful effects or little or no nutritional value.

Chapter 6 outlines *The TYTN Lifestyle* basics, including suggestions to customize the plan as per individual needs. In Chapter 7 you will learn what to expect while following the *TYTN Lifestyle* Plan. Chapter 8 includes several simple recipes and snack ideas. I share some final thoughts and suggestions in chapter 10, and a list of recommended resources in chapter 11.

The amount of carbohydrates you feel best eating will *ultimately need to be determined by you.* Next, let's look at what *is* included in *The TYTN Low-Carb Lifestyle* ~ Natures' own *prescribed way of eating and living.*

2 TYTN Staple Foods

1. **Animal flesh foods** - Any type of meats, fish, or fowl including a variety of cuts from beef, pork, chicken, turkey, other foul, mutton, wild game, buffalo, ostrich, etc..

2. **Products from animals** - Eggs, whole/full-fat and raw dairy products, including plain yogurts, ricotta cheese, 4% cottage cheese, sour cream, heavy whipping cream, half and half, whole milk, and other whole-fat cheeses, *as per your personal tolerance*[4]; organ meats, and products made from animals such as bacon and sausages providing they are of a better

---

[4]Lactose is a low-glycemic carbohydrate, or milk sugar found in mammal's milk created by the bonding of two different simple sugars, glucose and galactose. Lactase, a digestive enzyme, is needed to break the lactose bond apart to make the individual sugar molecules more easily absorbed. Most humans lose their ability to produce lactase by the age of 5. For this reason, many people may experience 'lactose intolerance.' Bacteria in the gut will ferment the lactose, creating lactic acid and gases which can lead to a variety of symptoms including gas, bloating, and diarrhea. Many people can still tolerate small amounts of dairy. Some people have a sensitivity to one or more of the dairy proteins in milk. These people may find that they well tolerate whole fat milk products like butter, heavy cream, sour cream, and possibly hard cheeses which contain minimal to no dairy protein.

quality, and free of excess sodium, sugars, and preservatives; natural fats from animals including beef tallow, non-hydrogenated pork lard, duck fat, butter, and bacon fat are used judiciously for cooking.

Emphasize whole cuts of meat over commercially raised processed meats.

Look for full-fat dairy products, such as sour cream or cottage cheese, that do not have added starches or gelatins. Sour cream should just be cream and enzymes, for example. Daisy brand out of Ohio is a good commercially available option.

3. **Leafy greens** - Any type of dark leafy greens including kale, collards, and beet, turnip, or mustard greens, lettuces, spinach, cabbage, dandelion leaves, arugula, bok choy, and fresh herbs.

4. **Other non-starchy vegetables** - The 'ABCs' of vegetables: asparagus, artichokes, beets, broccoli, Brussels sprouts, carrots, cauliflower, celery, and any other of your favorites (including those

that start with a different letter!): green beans, zucchini & other summer squash, and tomatoes and bell peppers which are technically fruits. *Eat only according to your desire and tolerance.*

5. **Fresh low-sugar/lower fructose fruits** - Berries, cherries, melons, citrus, and stone fruits, such as apricots, peaches, & plums; and green apples are generally best tolerated. Prioritize seasonal and local fruit, and eat according to your tolerance. Diabetics, and those with insulin resistance may need to keep fruit minimal, other than small amounts of berries and melons, at least initially.

6. **Fermented foods** - Naturally brined and (preferably homemade) fermented vegetables and pickles. Bubbie's is a good brand available commercially.

7. **Sea Vegetables** - Kelp, kombu, nori, dulce, arame, wakame, sea cucumber, etc. Add kelp or kombu to bone broth.

Notes:

Do your best to buy the best quality ingredients you can budget.

Here is our recommended order of priority:

1) Look for the best looking quality *you can afford*. The focus, at least initially, is on *eating according to your true nature* ~ the foods that will best help you improve your health and thrive. While I know many authors of paleo or ancestral health books are pretty emphatic about prioritizing organic, pasture-raised, grass-fed and finished animal products for the enhanced nutrition, we believe you will be fine ~ *better than fine* ~ if you just stick to the basics. Eat whole natural foods, rather than processed junk food. Most people are not able to budget 100% grass-fed animal foods. Let it be a goal, and do what you need to do, without feeling guilty.

2) Our next priority is to choose *locally produced* foods as much as able. We have a store that will feature 'Arizona raised' meats, which may cost a tad more, but is often much fresher looking. Whenever you can **grow or raise your own food**, that

is the ultimate best choice. If you can support a nearby farmer, that's a great option as well. At least purchase foods that are grown in your local bio-region, or country of origin as much as possible, rather than foods ~ especially perishables, like fruits and vegetables ~ from out of the country. Unless you are from or live near an area where tropical fruits including bananas, mangos, papaya, and others are grown, we recommend limiting them.

3) Okay, now I'll put in pasture raised, 100% grass-fed and grass-finished meats and animal foods. Grass-fed butter and cheeses like Kerrygold (from Ireland), Amish Roll Butter, and other local brands contain greater levels of vitamin A, important for skin and eye health, and conjugated linoleic acid (CLA) which has been found to support fat loss, among other benefits. If you are able, purchase locally produced eggs, and cheaper cuts of pastured meats. If your eggs are really pale yellow, you may want to try a different brand.

4) Purchase organic foods as able or desired. Integrated aquaponics and/or permaculture

growing systems that avoid mono-cropping practices, and therefore do not require the use of synthetic chemicals, fertilizers, and pesticides are actually preferred. Many who are growing food with more natural practices can not afford to go through the lengthy and expensive organic certification process. The majority of name-brand organic companies are owned by the bigger corporations, including Pepsi, Nestle, Coca-Cola, M&M Mars, General Mills, and Kellogg. Supporting local producers is preferred. As Don likes to say, *Don't major in the minors.* Labels can be misleading. Let your focus, at least initially, be on eating the right foods, organic or otherwise. Alternatively, consider growing at least some of your own fruits, herbs and vegetables, or raising animals for food, *as most people once did*, and as Don and I plan to do as soon as we are able.

5) Avoid purchasing refined, commercial plant oils. If using sunflower oil, **only** purchase if it is *high oleic, cold-pressed, and unrefined* as it is better quality, and higher in mono-unsaturated fats.

3 TYTN Supplementary Foods

Enjoy *With Caution*

1. **Starchy vegetables** - Winter squashes, including spaghetti, acorn, delicata, sweet dumpling, butternut, buttercup, kabocha, etc.; potatoes, especially red or purple skin potatoes, fingerlings, sweet potatoes, yams, etc.. Be sure to cut away the green parts and 'eyes' of potatoes which contain solanine, a glycoalkaloid, which can be toxic.

2. **Fruits** - Sweeter fruits, dried fruits, and those with higher levels of fructose, including apples and pears, can trigger those with fructose malabsorption.[5] If you

---

[5]Fructose malabsorption is a condition where one is not able to fully absorb fructose in the small intestine. The undigested fructose goes to the colon, where bacteria feeds on it, causing gas, intestinal swelling, abdominal distention, bloating, cramping, and possibly diarrhea. This is different than Hereditary Fructose Intolerance, HFI, which is caused by a deficiency of enzyme aldolase B, and leads to more severe symptoms, including vomiting, hypoglycemia, jaundice, and possibly kidney failure. Learn more: Amy Burkhart MD, RD, http://theceliacmd.com/2013/02/fructose-malabsorption-is-is-the-cause-of-my-tummy-troubles/, or Wikipedia, https://en.wikipedia.org/wiki/Hereditary_fructose_intolerance; and https://en.wikipedia.org/wiki/Fructose_malabsorption

are not sure how well you tolerate fruits, avoid all fruits for 2-4 weeks, then begin eating one serving per day to see how you respond. You may find you can tolerate half an apple versus an entire apple at one setting, for example. Otherwise, enjoy them as treats and if in good health as part of your total carbohydrate consumption.

3. **Nuts** - Pecans, hazelnuts, walnuts, pine nuts, pistachios, almonds, and macadamia nuts are the primary choices available within the United States or Europe. Nuts and seeds may be irritating to one's gut, and can be a source of inflammation, and skin break outs. If you suspect any symptoms being related to increased nut consumption, see how you feel eliminating them altogether for *at least* 2-4 weeks, then reintroduce them one at a time.

4. **Seeds** - Flax, hemp, chia, sesame, pumpkin and sunflower seeds are treated similar to nuts. Enjoy as tolerated. I have found that the more animal foods I eat, the less I crave nuts and seeds, and have observed them to be a source of intestinal discomfort, and skin break outs if consumed too frequently,

or in excess.

5. **Other fats & oils** - Oils from the above listed nuts, especially pecan and hazelnut are great choices; olives and good quality, single-source extra virgin olive oil (xvoo); macadamia nut oil; avocados and avocado oil; plain or toasted sesame oil, high oleic, cold-pressed and unrefined sunflower oil; coconut flesh, cream and oil. Emphasize whole food sources of fats, such as the fats intrinsic to animal meats, whole-fat dairy, and eggs; or butter, tallow, or other animal fats for cooking over extracted plant oils.

6. **Condiments** - Read labels! Look for low/ no added sugars, sodium, etc.; avoid if it contains dyes, soy oil, hydrogenated or partially hydrogenated oils, and any other unidentifiable ingredients or chemicals.

7. **Other** - Almond meal, coconut flour or flakes, coffee flour, nutritional yeast, herbs and seasonings that are preservative-free, real vanilla, natural preserves, and a little 85-100% dark chocolate can be enjoyed if not allergic.

4 FOODS TO MINIMIZE

Paleo diets typically exclude grains, grain products, and beans and legumes. We recommend for anyone with compromised digestive systems, allergies, a lot of phlegm and congestion, achey joints, high fasting insulin, or difficulty losing weight to *avoid all forms of these foods for at least one month* to determine if conditions improve.

1. **Whole grains** - Any variety of brown rice (short, medium, or long-grain, basmati, arborio, etc.) and other types of rice like wahini, black rice, or wild rice; millet; steel cut oats or whole oat groats; quinoa; teff; spelt; amaranth; barley; etc..

2. **Products made from whole grains** - Sprouted breads, or traditionally made sourdough or whole rye bread; whole-grain pasta; sprouted non-GMO corn tortillas. Gluten containing foods will need to be strictly avoided for anyone with known celiac disease (see below).

3. **Beans & products made with beans** Any type of beans, lentils, or legumes, preferably the smaller varieties; hummus and bean spreads; products made using chickpea or other bean flour; traditionally prepared soy products such as tofu, tempeh, miso paste or low-sodium, naturally brewed soy sauce.

4. **Nut butters** - Almond, macadamia, hazelnut, or pecan butters, or occasional peanut butter or tahini. Peanuts are actually a legume. Many people are highly allergic. Eat judiciously. Nut and seed butters are a dense fat, and generally used minimally, such as for baking special treats. Enjoy only according to your tolerance.

5. **Protein powders** - Whey, egg white, hemp, or possibly pea. These are highly refined and processed foods that are taken out of their whole state, and therefore not recommended as a TYTN primary or supplementary staple food. Use them sparingly, as needed.

6. **Treats** - High-fat, low-sugar traditional ice cream ~ preferably home made; home made lower-carb treats, chocolate that is not at least 85% dark, and anything you deem worthy of a splurge when out celebrating ~ only as appropriate for your level of health!

7. **Sweeteners** - Raw honey, real maple or birch syrup; low-glycemic, natural sugars, including stevia, Xlya, made from 100% North American hard-wood, popular in Europe; Swerve made from non-GMO ingredients derived from fruits and vegetables; monk fruit. Diabetics may want to avoid or greatly minimize the use of honey and syrup. Just because some of these sweeteners are 'safe' for diabetics or others on low-carb diets, doesn't mean they are good in large doses. *The dose makes the poison.*

Plant foods not edible in their raw state, such as grains, legumes, and even some nuts and seeds ~ while generally considered 'healthy foods' ~ are less desirable choices because of their higher susceptibility to containing anti-nutrients, and potential to cause digestive distress. It can be difficult to accurately determine how well these foods are tolerated until first *completely* eliminating them for *at least* one month, and then slowly adding them back, one at a time. The anti-nutrients, including phytates and fiber block absorption of important minerals, such as iron, zinc, and magnesium ~ the deficiencies for which may take time to be detectable.

I experienced increasing fatigue, dizzy spells, and other classic symptoms of iron deficiency *after* a few years of eating an entirely plant-based diet. Blood tests indicated normal range iron and B-12. My nails and lower eye lids were pale, I had dry skin and hair, and a pallor complexion. On paper, it looked like I was getting enough magnesium, zinc, and iron, but I now believe I was not properly assimilating these nutrients on a bean and grain-based vegan diet. I also had issues with constipation ~ despite my 'high-fiber' diet ~ and ongoing phlegm and sinus congestion, both of which finally began to resolve after eliminating grains, beans, and starches. If choosing to include these foods, cook them well, and test zinc levels with a liquid taste test, and iron levels with a blood test.

5 FOODS GENERALLY EXCLUDED

This next list includes foods that most of us should *avoid* the majority of time.

1. **Refined grain products** - Cookies, cakes, breads, bagels, donuts, pita bread, tortillas, noodles, and any other product made from refined flours, white flours, or wheat flour that is not 100% whole wheat; white rice. Small amounts of flour can be used here and there, but try to greatly limit your use.

2. **Gluten-containing products** - Any of the above items made with wheat, including 100% whole wheat, or any other product or condiment that contains any form of gluten (from wheat, rye, barley, and possibly spelt, kamut, and oats) for anyone who is *known celiac, has thyroid issues, is sensitive to wheat, has difficulty losing weight, constipation, or is in poor health.* Many people report feeling better from just eliminating wheat and gluten containing foods.

3. **Unhealthy fats** - Any fat labeled 'hydrogenated' or 'partially hydrogenated;' commercial plant oils including corn, canola, peanut, sunflower, safflower, or soy. Commercially made plant oils are often produced with solvents, are higher in omega 6 fatty acids, and can contain trans fats, all of which can cause increased inflammation and undermine health.

4. **Low-Fat/Non-Fat Dairy Products** - Avoid low- and non-fat milks and dairy products which are higher in carbohydrate, or sugar. Each person will have to discover their level of tolerance if choosing to consume dairy products. You may need to avoid *all* dairy foods, or only those higher in carbohydrates, or you may need to *limit* total consumption. Cultured or full-fat dairy products, such as yogurt, butter, ghee, heavy cream, cream cheese, and sour cream, with little to no dairy proteins, are typically best tolerated. Avoid synthetic cheeses.[6]

---

[6] Georgia Ede, MD has a comprehensive article about dairy, including what milk is comprised of, and the difference between an allergy versus a sensitivity to milk products on her blog, Diagnosis Diet, at http://www.diagnosisdiet.com/food/dairy/

5. **Snack foods** - Most crunchy, dry, salty snack foods, especially those high in sodium, hydrogenated oils, and refined sugars.

6. **Preservatives** - Foods with any type of synthetic or chemical-based ingredients, including food dyes. If you can't identify it, don't eat it.

7.**Pre-packaged foods** - For the most part, pre-packaged foods contain unwanted ingredients, unhealthful oils and sugars, and higher sodium than desirable per serving.

8. **Beverages** - Sodas and drinks made with synthetic sugars, high fructose corn syrup, caramel coloring, etc..

9. **Cereals** - Dry packaged cereals, especially those made from refined grains and sugars.

Generally speaking, *avoid the majority of foods found in the center aisles of the grocery store*, with the exception of canned tomatoes, tuna, sardines, mackerel, or salmon, and some condiments. Go right to the meat, dairy, and produce sections!

6 TYTN LIFESTYLE BASICS

Primarily consume foods from the list of primary staple foods to be *enjoyed freely*. Eat meats and eggs to satisfaction. Most people have an automatic limit to protein-rich foods. Once you have had enough of these nutrient-dense foods, having more at that meal will be unappealing. *Higher protein* low-carb diets have been found to be more satiating, and more effective at aiding weight loss then higher-fat, low-carb diets.[7]

Eat enough fat to feel satiated until your next meal. Don't skimp on healthy fats! If you don't consume adequate levels of *protein and fat*, you may end up craving more sweets or carbs, or feel more fatigued.

Fill in with the supplementary food choices as desired, and as per *your personal tolerance*. This primarily includes fruits, non-starchy vegetables, and greens, adding a little starchy

---

[7] *Relatively high-protein or 'low-carb' energy-restricted diets for body weight loss and body weight maintenance?* ScienceDirect-Physiology & Behavior, Vol. 107, issue 3, 10 Oct. 2012 https://www.sciencedirect.com/science/article/pii/S0031938412002806?via%3Dihub

tubers or winter squashes as needed. Eating more of those foods while transitioning to lower-carbohydrate intake may be helpful.

Foods, such as whole grains, whole grain products, and beans should be greatly reduced in your diet. It may be helpful to eliminate all grains and grain products, and beans and legumes for *at least* one month to determine how these foods are impacting your health and digestion.

We suggest making a mental commitment to avoid the foods to exclude outlined in Chapter 5 *for the most part*. These foods can be consumed out of necessity, or as a celebratory treat on occasion, however they are not supportive of human health. It's okay to use a little flour here or there to coat and pan fry a chicken breast, or to create a special treat. I don't believe in 'should-ing' on yourself as being too rigid is counter-productive.

Those in good health can certainly tolerate less healthful foods *on occasion* more than someone who is not, however, if you desire to be in the best health possible, why consume lesser quality foods? Be very honest with yourself, and maintain self-discipline. Focus on your goals to help overcome any urges for instant gratification.

We recommend consuming a **maximum** of 100g (grams) of carbohydrates per day *for most people, for the most part.* Men, athletes, and those in good health, or whom are trying to *gain* weight may be able to consume up to 150g. Petite women, older women, anyone who is desiring to lose weight, and less active individuals are advised to consume no more than 75g of carbohydrates per day. This is similar to the recommendation of limiting carbohydrate consumption to 72g per day found in *Life Without Bread.*

Adjust the total number of meals (including snacks), quantity of total calories, and percentages of macronutrients (protein, fat, and carbohydrates) according to *your current needs.* Your needs will vary depending on whether you are a male or female, your current weight and weight goals, energetic expenditure, and the condition of your health.

Basically, eat to satisfy your appetite, and *trust your true nature!*

When deciding what to eat, keep in mind that the most nutrient-dense foods will help you feel satiated quicker. Focus on eating these foods at the beginning of the meal. The most nutrient-dense foods are animal foods, especially eggs, red meats, and organs meats.

Many people may benefit from adopting time restrictive feeding practices, as outlined in Don's new book, *Primal Fasting*, now available. Having just two to three meals within a six to eight hour feeding window, with your final meal of the day 14-18 hours prior to breaking your fast the next day ~ at least a couple days per week ~ can greatly assist in reducing fasting insulin, and enhance weight loss.

Petite women and older women or those with weak digestion may prefer, at least initially, more frequent meal times. If you find that eating enough calories to satisfy your appetite at two to three main meals per day is too taxing to your digestive system, you may prefer to have at least three main meals and a snack, or four smaller meals each day. Emphasize protein with some healthy fats at each meal to help maintain blood sugar balance, and feel satiated until your next meal. A good ballpark is to consume around 75-125 grams, or 3-4 ounces of an animal protein source ~ such as 1-2 *Deviled Eggs*, or the amount of chicken, turkey, fish, beef, pork, etc. that will fit in the palm of your hand ~ at each of your *main* meals. Add enough fat to feel satiated, along with vegetables or a little fruit as desired.

Do your best to eat as seasonally, and locally as possible.

Try to support small local farms, and purchase the best quality foods that you can budget. Start by choosing at least one better quality and/or locally produced item at a time, such as eggs or dairy foods, for example.

Supporting those who are taking the care to feed their animals a species appropriate diet, and who practice more sustainable permaculture methods benefits all ~ you, the farmer, the animals, the soils, the greater community, and the local ecosystems.

The lower your intake of carbs, the easier to lose excess fat weight. This has actually been the preferred strategy until recent decades. The paradigm shift to emphasizing low-fat, higher carbohydrate diets and counting calories really got a foothold during the 1980s. For at least one hundred years prior, low-carbohydrate diets were found to be effective for weight loss, and managing diabetes. Since then, obesity, diabetes and other diseases, have risen dramatically. To fully grasp the ways that nutrition and dietary recommendations have been manipulated and polarized, I highly recommend reading *Good Calories, Bad Calories*, by Gary Taubes.

Keep your meals simple. Our meals were way more involved and elaborate when we were eating an entirely plant-based diet. A typical day of meals for us now may look like this: We usually start with our *High Protein Eggnog* post workout on the days we train, followed by a protein-rich meal soon after, such as chili, or *Stuffed Green Peppers*. The other mornings we typically have cooked eggs and either bacon, ham, or other meat. We may have some yogurt mixed with ricotta cheese, cottage cheese, or sliced ham with cheese and possibly a few raw veggies for a snack; and roast chicken, turkey, or beef with some bone broth for our final meal. If we have fermented cabbage or beets around, we have some with our roast. Otherwise, we have *Pan-Fried Cabbage* or other vegetables *as desired* with one of our main meals. If we are still hungry after a meal, we usually have tea, or a *Chicory Coffee* with a little heavy cream for dessert, or perhaps fresh berries with whipped or sour cream during the summer. After breakfast, I sometimes have 7-15g of 100% dark chocolate with my tea.

This is *your* life. Find the right balance for *you* to enjoy your life*, and* realize your health and weight goals. Our aim is to empower you to *trust your true nature*, and eat more *intuitively*, as opposed to strictly adhering to dogmatic or rigid ideologies or practices.

Learn to trust what your body is craving, and enjoy what you feel most drawn to, without over analyzing. Your body 'knows' what it needs, but your mind makes guesses and interpretations about what it craves.

Trust, but remain open and curious. You may eat mostly higher protein meals throughout the week, and then crave more fat on the weekend. You may really crave a lot of vegetables or fruit one day, and very little the next. Trust this. If you absolutely love bread, have some better quality bread here and there if it makes you happy, providing you are in good health, and adhere to the maximum carbohydrate recommendations.

If you have a history of chronic digestive discomfort, allergies, or skin disorders, it may surprise you to know that there are many seemingly healthy plant foods that may be the culprits. Our body does not produce enzymes to break down fiber, and plant foods do contain natural toxins that are mostly, but not always cooked out.

There are two lists of potential suspect foods to consider eliminating for 4-6 weeks, and then slowly reintroducing one at a time to determine tolerance. One is the list of FODMAP foods, and the other is a list of foods that are potentially high histamine triggers. These lists are pretty extensive. To avoid overwhelm, try following my simple suggestions on how to approach this, below.

7 WHAT TO EXPECT ON THE TYTN PLAN

You will need to experiment to determine which foods help you to feel your absolute best. This can take a little time, as your initial reaction to any change of diet will reflect the current health of your gut, which may need time to heal. Fiber swells because it soaks up water. It can actually cause a lot of problems, despite the prevailing belief that fiber is important to 'keep us regular.' A good book to read on this topic is *Fiber Menace*, listed in the resource section.

Give yourself enough time to acclimate to a higher protein and fat diet. Most people are consuming moderate to high-carb diets.

You may experience brief periods of increased fatigue, digestive discomforts, headaches, nausea, or even temporary weight gain in the early stages of transitioning to a low-carb diet. All of these things are normal.

When you begin to eat a much higher fat diet, you will also be changing your primary fuel source from glucose, the sugars formed from the break down of any carbohydrate foods, including vegetables and fruits (which also contain fructose), to fat. The fat can come from your diet, but it can also come from your own fat reserves ~ the ideal scenario ~ especially if weight loss, (or fat loss) are among your health goals.

Some people may choose to experiment with trying a very low-carbohydrate, high-fat (VLCHF) diet, consuming 50g *or less* of carbohydrates for at least 4-6 weeks. This is also referred to as a ketogenic diet. Ketones are produced by the liver and can be burned as fuel.

When you become adapted to burning fat for fuel, you will find that it is easier to go longer periods between meals.

Once you have burned up the fat from the foods you consumed, your body will automatically begin to use your *stored fat* to burn for energy ~ providing there is a net caloric deficit to your energy expenditures. If you keep eating more than enough fat to cover your energy output, and then some, you may not gain weight/fat as quickly as when over feeding carbohydrates, but you may also not be losing excess unwanted fat as readily either.

Many proponents of very low-carb or ketogenic diets make it sound like you can eat all the fat you desire, and suddenly become a fat-burning machine. I don't believe this is always the case.

Protein is needed for growth and repair, hormone production, and several other functions. Fatty acids, fat-soluble vitamins, *and cholesterol* also have a lot of important functions, including supporting the health of our brain, nerves, hormones, vision, skin, and much more, in addition to providing energy. Once you begin to give your body the raw materials it needs to do some (long overdue) healing and repair, you may find you *gain* a little weight before you actually begin to lose excess fat. And, if engaged in the right types of exercise, you may gain weight in the form of lean muscle mass, while losing fat ~ the ideal scenario.

In a nut shell, your body puts the raw materials of protein and fats to good use, allowing you to *seemingly* eat more without gaining fat, unlike when over feeding on carbohydrates which are not actually required by the body. The body can produce the amount of glucose needed for the brain from protein and fats.

While many believe that excess consumption of protein-rich foods, especially red meats is harmful, several studies indicate the contrary.

Protein and fats from animal sources are very satiating. When you have consumed enough essential amino acids and essential fatty acids ~ those required from food sources ~ the hormones in your brain will send signals, creating a feedback loop that will begin to shut your hunger down. That is why eating nutrient-dense proteins and fats help you to eat plenty without inadvertently over feeding, as is more typical when eating carbohydrate-rich diets.

The body is not able to obtain the same level of nutritional value from plant sources as these foods are less like our own tissues than animal foods. Plus, many plant foods have components that inhibit absorption of important nutrients.

When eating a carbohydrate-rich diet, the body relies on glucose for energy. There is a certain amount that is stored by the liver in the form of glycogen. This requires water for storage. The reserves can be used up quickly, depending on your energetic expenditure. When this happens, you may feel a dip in energy, or have other symptoms of low blood sugar until you eat your next meal.

The difference between being dependent on a continual feeding of glucose-containing foods, and being fat-adapted can be subtle, yet can also make a huge difference in your energy levels, moods, productivity, focus, and blood sugar balance.

It can be challenging initially to figure out which foods you feel good eating, and which foods you need to consume in smaller doses.

I personally found it helpful to greatly simplify my diet in the beginning to more easily determine which foods I can easily digest and assimilate, and which foods that I do not. Here is a summary of what I have discovered since adopting our TYTN diet:

- I feel best when I consume at least 25-30% of my total calories as protein, and roughly 55-60% as fat.

- I *do not* feel well when I eat a lot of high fibrous foods. I had ongoing constipation, abdominal distention, and many dizzy spells ~ to the point where I would have to brace myself before I would just drop ~ while eating a lower-fat, high-fiber vegan diet.

- I better tolerate the fruits that are at least equal in the ratio of glucose and fructose, preferably fruits higher in glucose than fructose, like strawberries, or cantaloupe. I am still experimenting, but I tend to best handle the equivalent of 3-6 oz. of berries (or up to 1 cup of strawberries) and *perhaps* 1/2 an apple or 25g of raisins in a day *at the most*.

- I seem to crave bacon (or ham) when I need to increase my sodium intake.

- I often eat 7-15g of 100% dark bakers chocolate after breakfast. Chocolate is a decent source of magnesium, and other nutrients. It helps me feel 'complete' with my meal.

- Getting adequate magnesium (versus higher fiber) has greatly improved my elimination. I suggest those who tend towards having constipation to try taking a 200-300mg dose up to three times daily with meals until elimination is more consistent. You can start with one per day, then two, then three, until you find the right dose without having very loose, sticky stools. Magnesium also improves absorption of calcium.

- When I eat the right amount, I leave the table feeling satisfied, without feeling overly full or bloated. If I do still feel hungry, I pause, and notice if the urge to eat passes. If not, I may have a *Chicory Coffee* with heavy cream as a sort of dessert, along with my 7.5-15g piece of 100% dark chocolate. That is usually just perfect. However, if when I pause, and I am no longer 'thinking' about food, I will wait a few hours, until the first impulse or thought of food arises again.

- I tend to eat within a 6-7 hour window of time ~ from 9:30-10:00, 12:30-1:00, and 3:30-4:00. Sometimes I do eat my last meal later. You will have to find your own sweet spot for the quantity of food per meal, and meals per day that helps you feel satisfied, to avoid inadvertently over feeding, crashing, or having cravings.

These are my personal discoveries. Some things may change over time. Pay attention to your patterns, and remain open, and patient with yourself.

About vegetables, there are people who are eating a 'zero-carb' diet, avoiding *all* added fruits and vegetables, and finding relief from allergies, and other difficult to diagnose conditions. Don has had tremendous success healing his decades long issue with psoriasis by eliminating most plant foods from the diet.

I mentioned FODMAPs and high histamine foods in the previous section. FODMAPs stands for **F**ermentable **O**ligosaccharides **D**isaccharides **M**onosaccharides **A**nd **P**olyols.

Here is a break down of what that entails:

- Fructose
- Lactose, found in dairy
- Fructans, found in wheat, garlic, onions, inulin, and more
- Galactans, found in beans and legumes
- Polyols, found in synthetic sweeteners, such as Sorbitol, Mannitol, Maltitol, Xylitol, and stone fruits such as avocados, apricots, cherries, nectarines, peaches, and plums

Foods high in histamines include alcohol, pickled foods (especially store bought vinegar pickles), some cheeses and dairy foods, certain fruits and vegetables, canned foods, shellfish, and some nuts and chocolate, to name a few. You can learn more about both of these groups and get lists at: HistamineIntoleranceAwareness.org., IBSdiets.org, and radicatamedicine.files.wordpress.com.

Rather than try to eliminate *all* the foods on either or both lists at once, here is what I suggest:

•Begin to simplify your diet, and reduce your total carbohydrate consumption.

•Eliminate all forms of refined sugars and processed foods first.

•Cut out all wheat products, and breads.

•Best would be to eliminate **all** grain and bean products for at least one month from the beginning, but if needing, do so if you do not have improvement *after* eliminating wheat products. Enjoy breads and grain products *only occasionally* as a treat, and/or only if you are certain that you tolerate wheat, gluten, and/or grains. If and when eating bread, traditionally fermented breads like whole grain sourdough are the best choice, followed by sprouted breads.

•Eliminate foods that are on the lists that you tend to *really crave*, or believe you *can't live without* ~ it's possible your gut bacteria is feeding on these foods! (Example: fruits, tomatoes, breads, nuts, or chocolate.)

•I suggest keeping a food journal and noting what you are eating plus your symptoms for as long as necessary. Look for patterns. *The 7-Day Food Mood Journal* is designed for this very purpose ~ to help people make the connection between the foods they eat, and their physical symptoms, and mental and emotional moods and energy fluctuations.

If the thought of eliminating a specific food seems difficult, it could indicate that it is a potential trigger. Eliminate it briefly to determine how you feel without it. Eat more protein and fat instead.

Our energy demands change daily, depending on mental and physical activity levels. When I first began a lower carbohydrate diet, I was pretty focused on eating plenty of fat. I was feeling better in many ways, yet not really losing excess body fat. After a couple months, I began focusing more on increasing my total protein. I fill in with enough fat to feel satisfied, only adding the amount of vegetables and fruits that feel appropriate at any given meal, which sometimes is none!

My primary health goals for switching to a low-carb diet included losing excess body fat while increasing lean muscle mass, reducing fasting glucose and balancing my blood sugar, improved digestion and elimination with less bloating and abdominal distention, and less phlegm congestion with a reduction in allergy symptoms. I believe I really aged myself while vegan ~ and several others concurred ~ so I also hope to recover lost youthful vitality and mental clarity, while lessening the premature aging, graying, and drying of my skin and hair. My vision diminished seemingly quickly as well.

Many of these began to show signs of improvement within the first six months following a higher-protein and fat, low-carbohydrate diet, including:

• The lower belly 'kangaroo pouch' seemed to melt away. I have an easier time digesting and assimilating the foods that I am eating. When I do eat something that I don't tolerate well, I will notice quickly, and tend to briefly experience abdominal distention, or a headache, otherwise, most of the abdominal discomfort has all but disappeared. My elimination may not be daily, but when I do go, it is much more effortless.

- My waist size went from 26 inches (or a bit more) at the end of over five years following a produce-rich, lower-fat, whole-foods plant-based, high-carbohydrate diet, to 25 inches, once I switched to a higher-protein + fat, very low-carb diet. I maintain a lower steady weight that is almost 5 pounds lower than my lowest weight while vegan. These are great indicators of having lost body fat, not just weight. Body recomposition takes time. I continue to pay attention to my inner cues, while remaining patient.

- My skin is MUCH softer. Even my elbows are no longer scaly!

- I have more color to my face again! My complexion was pale and ashen, a sign of blood deficiency according to traditional Chinese medicine (TCM) syndrome differentiation.

- My hair actually has a shine to it, and is less dull!

- My overall appearance is much brighter and healthier looking. I have had several people tell me as much, leading me to realize just

how tired and haggard I had been looking
while maintaining my 'healthy' too low-fat,
and nutrient-deficient, grain, bean and
vegetable-based macrobiotic diet.

- I no longer have weird twitchiness and
  nervous system imbalances that plagued me.

- My moods are much more even and upbeat,
  and I have much greater mental clarity.

- My blood sugar remains more balanced
  throughout the day. My energy and focus
  are more enduring. I can accomplish more,
  with less effort.

- I am no longer experiencing dizzy spells,
  nor any of the other miserable symptoms of
  low- (or high-) blood sugar.

- I easily train in a fasted state, recover
  quickly, and am having better results with
  muscular development.

- My body composition is finally getting
  closer to my long-standing ideal, which I
  struggled to realize on a low-fat, high-
  carbohydrate diet.

I believe that if you give *The Trust Your True Nature Low-Carb Lifestyle* a try, committing for at least three to six months, you will enjoy similar benefits. We have clients who have had similar success.

I've been so pleased with my results, and so much more convinced about the potentially negative impact of high-carbohydrate diets on human health, I can pretty confidently say "been there, done that, and *don't* need to (consume a high-carbohydrate diet) again!"

I believed that eating lots of 'antioxidant-rich' fruits and vegetables, along with the whole-grains and beans, while avoiding animal proteins and saturated fats would bring about all the results listed above. After over five years, I never achieved the long-term results I was looking for while being able to eat to satisfaction, without inadvertently over eating.

I previously took T. Colin Campbell's data ~ or at least the interpretation of it ~ as proof that eating excess protein was potentially dangerous. However, as Campbell himself teaches, it's important to closely examine all the components of how a research study is designed. Closer examination of his own research highlights how misleading studies can be. In his research he gave animals plant-based diets that were deficient in essential amino acids ~ an environment that is difficult to sustain. He found that tumors would not grow when the animals were eating these deficient diets, but did when given an isolated dairy protein with a complete amino acid profile. The problems here are: 1) He fed them an isolated protein, not a whole food, and 2) even if an amino acid deficient diet does prevent liver cancer, we can't thrive on diets lacking essential amino acids.

The truth is often buried if it counters invested interests, and the economic gains of those with the most to lose.

When I met Don, and began consuming a paleo diet, back in 2010, I had reached my all time highest weight (127 pounds), and developed the intense fibrocystic breast tenderness and fatty, enlarged breasts. That, along with ongoing constipation, allergies, and other issues led me away from animal-centered diets, believing the culprit of my poor health to be the animal foods and saturated fats ~ as is commonly taught.

I now realize it was a result of still consuming a higher intake of carbohydrates (primarily vegetables, greens, sweet potatoes, winter squash, and fruits, with some nuts and seeds) *along with* substantial portions of protein and fat. Higher carb + higher fat (and protein) was *not* a winning combination for me. I don't think it is a winning combination for most people. This combination caused my insulin to spike, and led to unwanted fat storage in the areas typical of one with metabolic syndrome ~ the lower abdomen, thighs, and buttocks, and my enlarged breasts.

Reducing my total carbohydrate consumption has helped me to resolve many of the health issues that have plagued me for much of my life while I continued to consume moderate to high-carbohydrate diets.

Here are some more points to consider to help *you* feel your best, realize your health goals, and energize your dreams while living the *TYTN, Low-Carb Lifestyle*:

1. Most people will do best when maintaining consistent, regular meal times, with each meal centering around some form of *protein-rich* foods.

2. It's okay to finish your meals and feel as if you could possibly eat *a little more*. Pause, then check in and see if you are still desiring more food. If so eat a bit more. Or, have a hot tea or *Chicory Coffee* for dessert. Otherwise, wait 2-3 hours, than eat again. *The TYTN Diet Plan* is about eating to satisfaction, and enjoying what you eat!

3. If you are practicing intermittent fasting, you will need to eat enough to feel satiated between meals. This generally requires higher quantities of healthy fats (from animal or plant sources), along with adequate protein.

4. Endurance athletes, such as long distant runners and cyclists, may find they perform better with an increased consumption of fat. There are studies indicating that people who are 'fat-adapted' do well with endurance sports. Pay attention to the health of your body

and joints, along with potential muscle wasting from not getting adequate nutrients, especially protein. You may like the documentary *Fat Chance* about a guy who cycled across Australia on a low-carb, high-fat diet, on DietDoctor.com.

5. Adjust your diet seasonally. Eat less fatty foods during the warmer months, more during the cooler season. Walnuts, for example, have a high fat content and are considered warming in Chinese medicine. Eating a lot of walnuts may generate too much internal heat if consumed in excess of what is appropriate for your condition constitution, and the season.

   Summer cooking methods are lighter and quicker: stir fries, grilling, boiling, broiling, and quick blanching, with more raw salads, vegetables and fruits, and cold beverages. Drink refreshing chilled teas like the *Rose Hips, Hibiscus & Chrysanthemum Tea* in section 7.

   Winter cooking methods add more heat, and are longer and slower: roasting, slow cooking, baking, more sautéed vegetables, less raw, and chai-spiced beverages made with warming spices, such as cinnamon, nutmeg, clove, allspice, and dried ginger.

6. If wanting to lose weight, I suggest having a higher protein focus. I'll share my secret formula: **PRO + FAT x 3**. Eat **3** meals, each with a **protein focus**, adding just enough **fat,** and one other item, like some fresh or fermented vegetables, or a little fruit for dessert. This way you will be having **3** main ingredients at each of **3** different meals, centered around a **protein** and **fat**. Of course, you can have more than 3 ingredients at a meal, more than three meals in a day, or just protein and fat if you desire. This is just a simple, easy to remember formula that works.

7. If you are trying to gain weight, you may try to increase your total calories, and total fat. Make sure you are engaging in an exercise routine, ideally weight training to ensure the weight you gain is primarily muscle, versus fat. Active people, and those trying to gain weight may feel better increasing total carbohydrates.

8. Cravings for sugars and carbs can indicate a need for consuming either more total calories, more consistent meal times, or more total protein and/or fat.

   When choosing carbohydrate-rich foods, focus on low-sugar fruit and non-starchy vegetables, followed by root vegetables and tubers, including sweet potatoes and winter squash. If eating grains, eat the whole form. Have some oats with whole-fat yogurt, nuts, a poached egg, sausage, or vegetables sautéed in olive oil, butter or ghee, as an example. Adding the fat will reduce the insulin spike; adding protein will make the meal more satiating and sustainable.

9. It is possible that some people may feel better eating higher protein with a *slightly* higher percentage of carbs in the form of fruits and vegetables, and a *slightly* lower intake of fat. Experiment to decide how you feel your best.

10. Don't forget if you have a lot of digestive issues or allergies, check out the Resources in Chapter 11 for online sources to learn

more about FODMAP foods, and high histamine foods.

To review, here is what I suggest if considering eliminating foods from either or both of these lists:

- Decide when you feel ready to dedicate 3-4 weeks to eating *very* simple meals with few ingredients.

- Focus on consuming mostly animal foods which are less likely to be triggers, with the possible exception of eggs and dairy foods for some.

- Eliminate those foods on the lists that you most often consume, especially those foods you feel strong cravings for. Keep track of your meals and symptoms to look for patterns.

- Once you begin to notice a lessening of symptoms, slowly add foods in one at a time to test for your reaction.

8 Meal & Snack Ideas & Recipes

I will start this section by sharing our very unconventional post workout fuel.

We spend about two hours doing our strength training routine, along with some stretching, three days per week. We have found the following supplements and protein drink to be ideal post strength-training, replenishing fuel:

After our morning exercise, we take (I should say chew) four Universal Nutrition Uni-Liver tablets, chasing it down with water, or a blend of 1/2 low-sodium vegetable juice and 1/2 water, plus 1 tsp. Carlson Labs Lemon Cod Liver Oil. We sometimes blend 1 tablespoon Now brand liver powder into the vegetable juice + water + oil combo instead, but the liver tablets are really not that bad tasting. They have stellar reviews on Amazon. One reviewer found that taking the liver tablets helped to reduce allergy symptoms.

Liver, contrary to what you may have heard, is truly the most super of super foods. It is very nourishing for your liver, builds blood, and is a good source of vitamin A, along with calcium, folate, and amino acids, the building blocks of protein. If you are feeling bold, or you do like liver, be sure to check out the *Liver, Onion & Tomato* recipe at the end of this section.

After this concoction, we often have eggs, and after training, we especially enjoy our super nourishing, *Protein-Rich Eggnog* ~ a blend of raw eggs with milk + heavy cream, or half and half, and possibly cinnamon, vanilla or cocoa powder, or a small amount of fruit.

The lecithin and choline in egg yolks are very important, and not found in similar quantities elsewhere. The fatty acids in the yolk actually help to *pull fat out* of the liver. Diets lacking in choline, and very low in fat can actually lead to non-alcoholic fatty liver disease.

I never thought I would consume raw eggs, but I am now an advocate, as I believe this drink, plus the liver tablets and cod liver oil are part of the reason I have had such an improvement in my skin, hair, and post training recovery.

Protein-Rich Eggnog:

3 eggs
1/2 - 3/4 cup+ liquid: 1/4 cup half & half + 1/4-1/2 cup water or previously brewed coffee or chai tea, or 1/2 cup of whole milk and 1-2 tbsp. heavy cream
1/4-1/2 tsp. cinnamon
1 tsp. vanilla ~ liquid or powder
Optionals: 2-3 tsp. unsweetened cocoa powder, 1/3 cup cantaloupe or 1/2 a peach, 1 scoop protein powder, &/or a pinch of stevia

Blend ingredients. Add more or less of whatever you like. You can use one less egg yolk, and sub 1/4 cup of egg white if you prefer a lower-fat version. I quite enjoy using a little coffee with the cocoa powder for my version of a protein-rich mocha!

Many people make smoothies using a variety of greens, fruit, and protein powders. While we have done so as well in the past, the above meal in a glass is pretty much the extent of our 'smoothies' these days. It's easy, and can be done in any commercial blender, like my old Osterizer. No fancy expensive blender, nor expensive protein powders or super foods required, however, using protein powder occasionally can be helpful. We just personally prefer not to rely on it.

While we often have eggs in some form for breakfast, we don't always. I have always considered all my meals to be appropriate any time of day, and hence I don't tend to distinguish between breakfast, lunch, and dinner. I more differentiate between a cooked meal versus a simpler snack. Sometimes, a bowl of chicken soup, or chili made with grass-fed beef hits the spot on a chilly morning!

Eggs are common breakfast fare for most people. They provide a great mix of protein, fat, potassium, and healthful nutrients as stated above. They also provide a satiating effect, helping you stave off hunger, and feel mentally focused and satisfied.

Eggs can be scrambled, fried, boiled, baked, or easily poached without taking too much time, or needing any fancy equipment. Here are a few egg recipes in case you need inspiration.

Easy Poached Eggs:

Spray a small, shallow bowl with an olive oil spray, or wipe with a little butter. Carefully crack 2 eggs , and/or 2 eggs + 1/4 cup of egg whites into the bowl.

Season eggs as desired. Whether I am poaching or frying eggs, I usually like to season them with a few grinds of Celtic Grey Sea Salt, cracked black pepper, dried parsley or oregano, and a sprinkle of paprika.

To poach, add a few inches of purified water to a pot that will fit one of those collapsable steamer baskets. (Ours does not have the piece of metal sticking up in the center like many do.) Bring to a boil. Place the basket in the pot, and the bowl of eggs in the basket.

Cover, and cook on medium heat until the tops of the whites are opaque and no longer liquid-y, but the yolk is still soft and runny, or to desired doneness, around 5-7 minutes.

Serve with whatever you like, including good quality, uncured bacon, sausage, or leftover steak reheated with onions and peppers and/or pan-fried greens or vegetables.

Fried Eggs:

Eggs can be fried on a good quality, non-stick pan without any added fat. However, sometimes adding fat can increase the satiety at breakfast time. Add a little butter, or cook in the fat after first cooking bacon.

Cook eggs on a medium heat until desired doneness, or quickly flip for 'over easy.' They can also be basted using a big spoon to collect the bacon fat, and pouring it over the egg yolk. Lift the pan up slightly so that you can capture the bacon grease. Yes, you now have permission to baste your eggs in bacon fat!

Alternatively, cook eggs in a cast iron skillet in a little butter, cover the pan, and cook on medium until the top of the egg is an opaque, almost pink color.

Serve eggs as desired, with a meat of choice, including *My Simple Ground Beef & Zucchini* (recipe below), or with sautéed spinach, or other greens. Eggs are also good with fresh or sautéed tomato and *Parsley or Basil Pesto.*

Be sure to check out my simple and delicious *Baked Eggs w/ Turkey & Smoked Cheddar* video recipe on my YouTube channel.

Bacon, Tomato, Eggs & Basil:

2+ slices of bacon, pork belly, or ham, torn into 2-3 inch pieces
1 Roma tomato per person, sliced
2-3+ eggs per person
Sea salt, cracked black pepper, & pinch of red pepper flakes
Several fresh basil leaves, cut into smaller pieces

I prepare this on our round, non-stick griddle pan. Place bacon or ham on a pan or griddle set to medium heat. Cook a few minutes until it begins to brown. Turn over. Add tomatoes around the perimeter of the pan, and move the bacon or ham over to rest on top of the tomatoes, roughly, to create space for the eggs.

Pour the eggs in the center. Season with sea salt, pepper, dried parsley, and a pinch of red pepper flakes. Cook until the whites turn opaque, but the yolks are still runny. Sprinkle basil all over on top.

My Favorite Super Soft Scrambled Eggs:

Amounts are per serving.

2-3+ eggs
Splash cold water
2-3 tsp. butter ~ great with salted Amish Roll Butter! (or any good quality/grass-fed butter)
Sea salt, pepper
Optional: 1 oz. shredded cheese of choice ~ grass-fed cheddar, whole-fat mozzarella, etc.

Whisk the eggs with a splash of cold water *very well.* Warm a skillet on medium heat, and add butter. Once melted, add eggs. Season with salt and pepper.

After the first couple minutes, use a wooden spatula to push the eggs towards the center.

Keep scraping, and turning the heat down as it gets more cooked. If using cheese, add about half way into the cooking. Cook and scrape on low until *just* cooked through. Serve as desired.

Variations:
- Add diced onion, zucchini, mushroom and/or bell pepper to the skillet a few minutes before adding eggs. Cook as above. If using vegetables, cook them in 1-2 tsp. of olive oil first, then add 1-2 tsp. butter prior to adding eggs.
- Season eggs with a little turmeric and/or nutritional yeast.
- **French Eggs:** Sauté 2-3 sliced scallions or a leek & a clove of garlic in 1 tbsp. butter. Add eggs. As the eggs begin to cook, add 1+ ounce whole-fat cream cheese, goat cheese, or 1/4 cup cottage cheese. Cook as above.

Egg Pizza:

2-3 eggs per serving
Splash cold water
Sea salt, pepper
1-1.5 tsp. unsalted butter

Vegetables: Diced zucchini, red bell pepper, red onion, mushroom, and/or cut up greens of choice
Fresh or dried basil and/or oregano
1-2 tsp. olive oil

Prepare eggs by whipping well in a bowl with the splash of cold water, and set aside.

Warm a skillet, and add olive oil. Add vegetables, a little sea salt, and fresh or dried herbs. Sauté 3-4 minutes, until tender. Remove from pan.

Add butter. Once melted, add eggs. Season eggs with sea salt and pepper. Let eggs cook undisturbed for a couple minutes. When the edges begin to set, use a spatula to scrape around the edges, lifting to let the uncooked eggs get underneath. Repeat this around the pan.

When mostly cooked, add vegetables on top of the eggs. The eggs may still be runny at this point. Make sure heat is fairly low to not burn the bottom. Cover, and let cook a few minutes. Turn heat off, but leave cover on for another minute or two to prevent sticking.

If you have an oven-proof pan, you could also finish cooking uncovered in the oven. Top with grated cheese first if desired.

Vary it by using pan-fried diced ham, pancetta, sausage, chicken or turkey with spinach or other greens, tomato, or vegetables.

I recently read a newsletter from someone marketing a cookbook featuring breakfast foods for those on a paleo diet. There was a lot of build up to her story, about being unhealthy, trying lots of diets, then finding the paleo diet, and finally getting better. She was all excited at first to eat eggs and bacon.

Many people feel this way when first learning that eating eggs cooked in bacon fat or butter can actually be part of a healthy diet.

What I found interesting was the rest of the story. She quickly turned bored of her egg breakfasts, and spent a long time researching and experimenting with other online recipes, much of which she didn't really like. Her 'ah ha' moment came when she realized that breakfast foods did not *have to* be centered around eggs when foregoing the other standard breakfast items, such as cold or hot cereal, or a muffin on the run.

I've always tended to think outside the box, so I never needed to spend years coming up with recipes for alternatives to eggs. I find eggs very satisfying and delicious, and I vary them as I feel inclined, mostly by varying what I eat with the eggs.

I also enjoy eating leftovers for breakfast with or without eggs, whether steak that I quickly re-heat in the pan with a little bacon fat, left-over *Stewed Chicken*, below, or a big bowl of *Bone Broth* with *Slow Roasted Beef.*

Her story about her lengthy time spent researching recipes enabled her to offer her book at a much discounted rate, from what was hyped up to be of a near $100 value otherwise. $100 for a recipe book???

Personally, as I see it, the more people realize that these traditional staple foods of our *once healthy* Western diet are *the most nourishing and nutrient-dense foods*, and that the manufactured foods that have only been around since the Industrial Revolution are *robbing us of our health*, the sooner we can begin to reverse the nation-wide trends of obesity, diabetes, and premature crippling and aging. Wouldn't you like to realize your full physical and mental potential, retaining full functioning as you age? We all benefit from a healthier populace ~ that is except those who profit from our being sick.

Aside from eggs, meals can center around your animal protein of choice with a little bone broth and/or vegetables, or a high-protein or whole-fat dairy, such as 4% cottage cheese or yogurt ~ plain, or with berries, cinnamon, and/or a few chopped pecans.

The simpler the meals, the better, especially when healing a dysfunctional digestive system. If you are not in the mood for a lot of vegetables, don't have much. I no longer believe you need to have *any*, but I know it will take time before more people are on board with eating a carnivorous diet with few to no plant foods. *The TYTN Low Carb Lifestyle* allows everyone to make choices according to *their own needs, cravings, and personal evolution*. There are many people eating mostly just meat and eggs, and some that are eating mostly whole-fat dairy foods who are reporting improved energy and health. You won't really know how you feel eating mostly just animal foods until you try!

If you do still crave or enjoy greens, have a salad as your main entrée, topped with plenty of protein ~ grilled or cooked chicken, turkey, steak, taco meat, salmon, or ahi tuna. You may want to try the *Radish Greens Pressed Salad*, below. Squeezing the greens and vegetables for a couple minutes improves their digestibility, and brings out their full flavor.

Among my favorite meals is a perfectly grilled or pan-fried sirloin steak with sautéed onions and mushrooms. Also good with the *Radish Greens Pressed Salad.*

Grilled Sirloin Steak with Sautéed Onions & Mushrooms: *We often use petite sirloin steaks, or chuck steaks with great results, but use your favorite.*

1 125-175g(+) steak per person
Extra virgin olive oil (xvoo) ~ for the steak

Sea salt & pepper
Optional: garlic powder &/or cumin
1 sweet or yellow onion, sliced
Several mushrooms of choice, sliced
Butter &/or xvoo for cooking
Dried oregano

Prepare steaks. Place on a plate, pat dry if needed, drizzle with oil, then season with sea salt, pepper, and optional garlic powder, and/or cumin. This can be done ahead of time, and left in the refrigerator until 10-20 minutes prior to cooking.

When ready, prepare vegetables. Warm a pan. Add 2-3 tsp. olive oil and/or butter. (The oil prevents the butter from over heating and turning brown.)

Add onions, and let cook a few minutes. Add mushrooms, and season with sea salt, pepper, and a little dried oregano.

If this mixture begins to dry out, add another teaspoon or so of butter, or a bit more oil. Let cook on medium-low with the lid slightly ajar until soft and browning.

Grill steak on an outdoor grill, cast iron grill pan, or a non-stick griddle which you can lightly brush with a little butter. Grill or pan-fry until nicely browned, or you have grill marks, turning 90° for the cross marks.

Flip, and turn heat to medium. Continue to cook until desired doneness. We like it cooked to about medium-rare. I can tell by the feel when it is cooked to our liking. Medium-rare will have a little give when pressed with a finger, without being too mushy.

Once cooked, let sit for a couple minutes before cutting, then slice thin, and enjoy!

Radish Greens Pressed Salad:

1 bunch radish greens, cleaned and chopped
4 radishes, diced
1/4 red onion, or 2 scallions, diced
1/2 cucumber, diced
1 fresh tomato, diced
1+ tbsp. xvoo, or other oil, such as hazelnut, pecan, avocado, toasted sesame oil, or a blend
A few splashes balsamic vinegar
Sea salt

Place greens and vegetables in a salad bowl. Drizzle with oil of choice. Place index finger on top of vinegar bottle to shake out several drops of vinegar. Season with a little sea salt.

Using your hand, squeeze contents several times to help break down the vegetables. This will help improve digestion, and bring out the flavor of the vegetables.

Have fun, and experiment with some of our own American made oils like hazelnut and pecan which have a good fatty acid profile. Use whatever greens and veggies you like.

Vinaigrette Dressing:

1 tbsp. - 1/4 cup xvoo, or other nut oil
About 1/3 as much balsamic vinegar
Pinch sea salt & pepper
Pinch dried thyme, lavender, or herbs de Provence
Pinch stevia or 1/2-1 tsp. real maple syrup
1/2-1 tsp. dijon mustard

Shake ingredients in a jar. Adjust oil, vinegar, and salt to taste. Use what you need, save the rest for another day.

Sautéed Zucchini, Onion & Tomato:

1-2 tbsp. xvoo
1 large sweet or yellow onion, sliced
2-4 cloves garlic, minced
3-4 zucchinis, cut in whatever shapes you like
2 Roma tomatoes, diced
Sea salt, pepper, & dried oregano

Warm a pan, and add oil. Add onion, and
sauté 5-7 minutes, until the onion begins to
soften. Add remaining ingredients. Let cook
on medium-low until zucchini has softened.
Serve with grilled steak or chicken, or prepare
with sausages for another alternative.

Slow Roast Cooking Method: *Roast once,
eat at least twice, or thrice!*

We have a new routine on the weekends ~
'Slow Roast Sunday'. We love the slow roast
preparation method, as it's practically fool-
proof, and it provides us with a few days
worth of quick meals for the start of our work
week. I wrote in a blog post about placing a
beef brisket *on top of* a roast in our Le
Creuset Dutch Oven, cooking a fattier cut on
top of a leaner cut at the same time.

The slow cooking method is considered safer, and creates really tender, flavorful roasts, ribs, shanks, and other cuts of meat.

Marinate meats first, time permitting. For beef roasts, drizzle with a little balsamic vinegar, and rub coarse sea salt, and optional garlic and rosemary or smoked paprika all over the roast. You can alternatively cut thin slits all around the meat to add sliced pieces of fresh garlic clove. Or just rub in salt and pepper.

Pre-marinate pork or poultry in a little apple cider vinegar, or fresh citrus, then rub all over with sea salt, white pepper, and any other desired seasonings: rosemary, or dried ginger with a little ground star anise, allspice, or Chinese five spice are good on pork; dried thyme, sage, and herbs de Provence are great on poultry; rosemary, garlic, and/or sumac is good on lamb.

For beef roasts: Sauté sliced onions in a little bacon fat, or butter in a Dutch oven pot. Add roast, and any other vegetables desired.

For pork roast: Slice an apple, and place pork roast on top.

Our preferred method is to preheat the oven to 500°. Place roast (or turkey breast) in the oven uncovered for about 10 - 20 minutes ~ about 5 minutes per pound. This will sear the outside, and create a nice outer crust.

Turn heat down to 200°, and let it roast for about 6+ hours for a 2-3 pound roast. The internal temperature should be about 140° ~ a little higher or lower, depending on the type of meat, and your desired level of doneness.

We roast meats uncovered, but you can add a cover once seared. The final texture will be a little different. Try both and see which you prefer. Dryer meats may do better covered.

For slow roasted poultry parts, such as turkey thighs: Season with sea salt, pepper, dried thyme, sage and rosemary. Place in a baking dish on top of sliced green apple. Add a few thin shavings of butter on top of the parts, getting some underneath the skin.

Cook uncovered at about 450° for the first 15 minutes, then reduce heat to 200°, and roast as above, until the internal temperature is 160°. Super delicious!

For turkey breast: Do a semi-dry brine first. Squeeze the juice of about half an orange on a turkey breast, then rub coarse sea salt, and herbs de Provence, thyme, sage, and/or rosemary all over. Lift some skin to rub salt on the flesh. Let sit uncovered in your fridge overnight. When ready, preheat oven to 500° and roast for about 15 minutes, until the skin begins to brown. Turn low, and roast as above. The meat will be moist and tender.

If using a slow cooker, cook roasts on high for the first hour, then reduce heat to low and let it cook all day, or overnight.

I used to prepare **lamb shanks** this way while in school studying acupuncture and Chinese medicine. They are delicious cooked in a crock pot with canned tomatoes, a little red wine, and a few prunes and/or chopped sweet potato or rutabaga for sweetness. I would also add a piece of dang gui (angelica root) which has a sweet, slightly licorice-y flavor, and helps build the blood.

Basic Burgers:

When able, look for locally raised meat made from cows that were grass-fed (GF) and grass-finished ~ pastured for their entire life.

1+ lb. ground beef
Sea salt, cracked pepper, garlic powder
Bacon fat and/or butter, optional

Using hands, shape meat into equal-sized, 4 oz. patties. Season, then fold the patties so that the seasoning ends up in the middle. Add more seasoning to the top side. Warm a grill pan, or non-stick griddle, to just above medium heat. Place burgers on pan, seasoned side down. Season the other side, and let cook until nicely browned. If using a grill pan, turn 90° to create the criss cross shaped grill marks. After a couple minutes, flip.

Turn the heat down to medium-low, and let the meat cook another 5+ minutes to desired doneness. The burger should feel somewhat firm, with a little give when pressed on the top with a finger.

Cover the burger if needed to help it cook to desired temp without drying out.

If you want to increase the fat, add a little bacon fat or butter to the pan, either before beginning, or after flipping the burger. Pour on top of burgers when serving. If monitoring fat intake, cook without added fat on the grill, or non-stick griddle pan.

If adding cheese, add the last couple minutes of cooking. Cover and cook on medium-low until cheese is melted, and burger is cooked.

Serve with sautéed onions and mushrooms, sliced tomato, bacon or avocado, and any of your favorite condiments.

For extra snazzy sautéed onions, stir in 1 heaping teaspoon of whole grain mustard once onions have softened, and cook until nicely browned.

My Simple Ground Beef & Zucchini:

.5-1 tbsp. xvoo, beef tallow, or bacon fat
1-1.5 lb. 85% lean or GF ground beef
1 lg. onion, chopped
Several mushrooms, sliced or chopped
2 cloves garlic, minced
3 zucchini, quartered lengthwise, then
chopped
1 red bell pepper, chopped
1-2 fresh tomatoes, chopped
Sea salt
Generous amount of ground cumin
Chili powder and/or pinch of cayenne pepper

Warm a large skillet and add olive oil. Add
onion, and let cook for a few minutes before
adding mushrooms and garlic. Season with
salt. Stir and cook a couple more minutes,
until the onion begins to turn translucent.

Add the remaining ingredients. Using a
wooden spatula, break up the meat. Cover,
and let it cook on medium-low for about 10
minutes or until vegetables are soft.

Variations:

- This is also good made with ground lamb or turkey breast.
- Add fresh fennel, or ground fennel seeds.
- Add chopped fresh tomatoes.
- Add a can of fire roasted petite diced tomatoes, or green chilis.

Matesz Meatloaf: *I suggest making extra for leftovers!*

2-3 lb. 85% lean (GF) ground beef
2 eggs
1 onion, diced
1 lg. green bell pepper, diced (*I've so come around to loving green bell peppers, especially in this meatloaf!*)
1/2-1 bunch parsley, finely chopped
About 1 tbsp. coarse sea salt, less if fine
1+ tsp. white &/or black pepper
Other herbs or spices desired, such as ground fennel, oregano, smoked paprika
Optional: 1-2 tsp. sweet pepper relish, sweet pickle relish, or 1 tsp. Xyla or a couple pinches of stevia

Prepare 1-2 baking loaves, depending on how much you make. I usually wipe it with a good amount of beef tallow.

Preheat oven to 425°. Place all ingredients in a large bowl, and use your hands to work until nicely combined. Pat the meat mixture into the loaf pan(s). Bake at 425° for the first 10 minutes, then reduce to 275-300° and bake for about one hour. Top with barbecue sauce, such as either of those below, then return to the oven for another 10-15 minutes. Let cool a couple minutes before serving.

Simple Barbecue Sauce:

1/3-1/2 cup ketchup or tomato paste or sauce
1 tsp. dry yellow mustard (or ginger)
1/4 tsp. sea salt or 1/2 tsp. naturally fermented, wheat-free soy sauce
1+ tsp. Xyla, honey, maple syrup, or black strap molasses ~ choose according to your health needs & preferences
Optional: A few drops of liquid smoke, or .5 tsp. toasted sesame oil

Combine ingredients in a small bowl. Take a fork or knife and make a few holes or slits through the top of the meatloaf so a little of the sauce will penetrate. Cover the top of the meatloaf with sauce, then return to oven for another 10-15 minutes.

Modified NeanderThin Barbecue Sauce:

The original recipe also includes juice of an orange, but I preferred it without. The sauce gets better as it ages, and will keep up to a week in the fridge.

2 cloves garlic, minced
2 tbsp. onion, finely chopped
2 tbsp. bacon fat
1 tsp. chili powder
1 tsp. ground or crushed rosemary
1/2 tsp. ground coriander seeds
1 tsp. ground ginger
1 6-oz. can tomato paste
1/2 cup water, +/-
6 oz. apple juice
About 1/2 tsp. liquid hickory smoke, optional
A pinch or two of stevia, optional
Sauté garlic and onion in bacon fat over medium-low heat until tender, 5-10 minutes.

Add spices. Stir, then add remaining ingredients. Stir until well-blended. Cover and simmer over low heat for 5-10 minutes (30 minutes according to the original recipe) to let flavors blend.

Place sauce on meatloaf as described above. This sauce is also good on ribs.

Variations:
• Stuff the raw meat mixture into hollowed out, previously steamed bell peppers. Place in a Dutch oven pot. Top with tomato sauce, and bake at 350° for the first 10 minutes, then 300° for about one hour.
• Make *Cabbage Rolls*: Boil a cabbage to separate leaves. Cut down outer rib. Roll meat inside cabbage leaves, and bake as above, layered with tomato sauce, or simmer in a deep pan on the stove.
• Try the *Low-Carb Stuffed Peppers* recipe from my website.

Slow-Roasted Ribs:

1 full rack of baby back or spare ribs
Apple cider vinegar
Sea salt, white or black pepper, and garlic powder
Liquid smoke

NeanderThin Barbecue Sauce

Preheat oven to 500°.

Place ribs in a roasting pan or baking dish. Rub sea salt, pepper, liquid smoke, and any other desired spices, such as smoked paprika, garlic powder, or cumin into the ribs. Place in the oven for 15 minutes to begin to brown the meat, then reduce temperature to 200° and let roast for 6-7 hours.

Remove from heat, and add sauce. Let roast another 20 minutes or so. The meat should be fall off the bone tender.

If while cooking, it gets too brown, loosely cover with a foil tent.

Perfectly Cooked Pork Chops: *If you marinate lean pork chops and chicken breast in an acid before cooking, it will help to break down the muscle fibers, and maintain it's moisture while cooking.*

1+ center cut, boneless pork chop per person
Juice of 1 lime
Olive oil &/or unsalted butter

Sea salt, cracked pepper & garlic powder

Place pork chops in a large ziplock bag. Add lime juice. Seal bag, and massage chops to evenly distribute the lime juice. Let sit for at least one hour, preferably overnight.

When it is time to prepare, pat the chops dry. Season the top side with sea salt, pepper, and garlic powder. Warm a grill pan, or a non-stick griddle, or stainless steel pan on medium, or a little higher heat. Add 1-2 tsp. each of olive oil, *and* butter. Place chops on the pan, seasoned side down. Season the other side that is now facing up.

Let chops cook until nicely browned. Flip chops, then turn heat down to about medium-low. Cook until an inner temperature of about 135-140º. Serve with *Sautéed Spinach, Onion & Tomato*.

Sautéed Spinach, Onion & Tomato:

1-2 tsp. each xvoo & butter (or either/or)
1/2 -1 onion, sliced
Several mushrooms, chopped
1-2 cloves garlic, chopped or minced

Sea salt and cracked black pepper
1-2 Roma tomatoes, chopped
Pinch each of red pepper flakes, & basil or oregano
1/2-1 bunch of spinach, cleaned & coarsely chopped

Warm a pan, and add oil &/or butter. Add onion, and let cook for a couple minutes before adding mushrooms, and garlic. Season with salt and pepper. Add tomato and the remaining desired spices and herbs, stir, then add the spinach. Cover, and let cook on medium to medium-low until spinach has cooked down.

This makes a nice sauce which further boosts the juiciness of this dish! Prepare extra, and let leftover pork sit in the 'saucy' vegetables overnight. Reheat, covered the next day.

Ginger Soy Marinated & Roasted Chicken or Turkey Parts:

4+ chicken or turkey thighs, drumsticks or wings
1/4 cup toasted sesame oil or xvoo

2 tbsp. low-sodium natural soy sauce, or liquid aminos
Juice of half an orange, or 1 lemon or lime
1 inch piece of ginger, grated and squeezed or .5-1 tsp. dried ginger or dried yellow mustard
A few pinches of stevia, or 1-2 tsp. Swerve, Xyla, or natural sweetener of choice

Place chicken or turkey in a big bowl, or ziplock bag. Combine marinade ingredients in a small bowl. Pour over chicken/turkey and massage all over until evenly coated. Let sit at least one hour to overnight in the fridge.

When ready to cook, preheat oven to 400°. Place parts in a shallow baking dish or roasting pan with a little of the marinade. Roast for about 50-60 minutes, turning every 20 minutes.

For a more moist and tender chicken or turkey, roast for 10 minutes uncovered, then cover with foil, turn the heat to 275-300° and let it cook for 1+ hour, until the meat is tender, and easily pulls away from the bone.

Variations:
•Vary the marinade by substituting apple cider vinegar, or balsamic vinegar for the citrus. Season with rosemary, thyme, sea salt and pepper instead of ginger.
•Vary the marinade by combining about 1/2 cup of apple juice, with 1 tsp. each dry ginger, and turmeric, along with 1/2-1 tsp. sea salt. When ready to cook, place in a baking dish or roasting pan, and add some or all of the marinade to the pan, so you have about 1/4 inch of liquid. Roast as above.

Polish-Hungarian Inspired Chicken, Sauerkraut & Tomato: *We both enjoy this dish quite a bit. The Le Creuset Dutch Oven works well, otherwise use any glass or ceramic baking dish, and cover with aluminum foil. Hearty and warming!*

1-2 large onions, sliced in thick wedges
1/4 cabbage, chopped or sliced
2-3 bone-in chicken breasts, with skin
1 cup sauerkraut + brine water
1 can petite diced tomatoes (can be fire roasted)

Dried or fresh thyme, rosemary, and/or oregano and basil
Optional: A few pieces of ham *fat*, ham, or a slice of bacon; sliced pieces of liver
Preheat oven to 400°.

Place onion wedges in bottom of cooking pot. Add chopped cabbage, then chicken breasts. Pour sauerkraut, and some brine liquid on top of the chicken, then add the tomatoes. Season as generously as desired with oregano and basil. Place ham/ham fat or bacon on the very top. If adding liver, place on top of the onions so they soak up the juices while cooking.

Cover and place in oven. Cook for up to 10 minutes at 400° before turning the temperature to about 275°. Let roast for around 2 hours, or until the chicken breast meat can be easily torn apart with a fork. Dish out and enjoy!

Notes: If you don't have sauerkraut on hand, add some broth instead, and season chicken with sea salt. Store bought pickles are typically made with vinegar, so if using, only use a *little* of the juice.

The sauerkraut I usually prefer is our own homemade fermented cabbage made in a simple salt brine. I like to keep the brine liquid, even when out of the fermented cabbage to use the liquid for cooking this delicious dish.

Variations:
- Sauté the onions in bacon fat right in the cooking pot prior to adding the chicken. If using liver, add to the onions to quickly sear before adding remaining ingredients.
- Try making this with a mix of chicken ~ breasts, thighs, or drumsticks ~ and polish sausage or kielbasa.
- Add celery, carrots, mushrooms, Brussels sprouts, turnips, or chopped beets if desired.
- Substitute olives or sun-dried tomatoes if needed in lieu of sauerkraut.
- Use this same cooking method for any other meat and vegetable combination you can imagine, such as stew meat or lamb shanks. Cooking times may vary.

Pesto Chicken or Pork:

2-4 boneless, skinless chicken breasts, or lean pork chop

Juice of 1/2-1 lemon or lime
1 tbsp. xvoo + 1 tbsp. butter
Sea salt and pepper
1/2-1 cup either *Parsley Almond* or *Basil Pesto Sauce*, below

Place chicken breasts on a cutting board, and slice into half the thickness. It may be easier to cut when slightly frozen. Place in a ziplock bag, and add lemon or lime juice. Let marinate for 1 hour to overnight.

When ready to cook, pat dry, and season both sides with sea salt & pepper. Warm a pan on just above medium heat. Add oil and/or butter. Let cook until evenly browned, then turn. Cook until nicely browned on the second side.

Add pesto sauce, turn to medium-low, cover, and simmer for 3-5 minutes, until the chicken is tender, juicy and cooked through. You could also bake the chicken at 300° with the pesto sauce if desired.

Parsley Almond Pesto:

1/2 bunch of parsley, big stems removed

Juice of 1/2-1 lemon
1/4 cup almonds
1 tbsp. nutritional yeast
1 clove garlic
Pinch each of sea salt & pepper
1tbsp. ghee or butter, melted
1/4 cup xvoo, hazelnut oil, or pecan oil

Place parsley and almonds in a food processor, and pulse until almonds are fairly well chopped, without becoming a paste. Add the rest of the ingredients, up to the oil. Turn processor on, and slowly pour oil in. Scrape sides, and blend until well combined. Adjust flavor as needed.

Basil Pesto:

4 cups basil, loosely packed or a mix of basil & parsley
Juice of 1/2+ lemon
1-2 small cloves garlic
2 tbsp. nutritional yeast, or parmesan cheese
1-2 re-hydrated sun-dried tomatoes plus 2-3 tsp. soaking liquid
Pinch each sea salt & black pepper or red pepper flakes
1/4 cup xvoo, hazelnut oil, or pecan oil

Place ingredients except oil in a food processor. Add oil while processing, as above. Blend until well combined. Adjust flavor and seasoning as needed.

Kielbasa, Onion & Beet Greens:

1/2 sweet or yellow onion, coarse chopped
1 garlic clove, chopped or minced
1 pkg. kielbasa, pork or turkey, sliced
1 bunch beet greens, cleaned and chopped
2 Roma Tomatoes, diced
~ 1 tsp. xvoo + 2-3 tsp. bacon fat, or cooking fat of choice

Warm a pan, and add fat. When hot, add onion. Cook for a minute or two before adding garlic.

Add kielbasa to the onions. Let cook at medium heat or a little higher, shaking pan, or stirring to brown, but prevent burning. After about 5 minutes, add the beet greens and tomatoes. Cover and let cook on low for another 7-10 minutes.

Liver, Tomato & Onion Variation: *I know liver is not everyone's favorite, but it is super* *nourishing. According to traditional Chinese medicine (TCM), pork liver nourishes the yin ~ the nutritive essence or lube that keeps us young and vital. Try this with pork, beef, or chicken livers. Make sure to purchase organic or grass-fed. Preparing this in a cast iron skillet will further boost the iron absorption.*

2-3 tsp. bacon fat
25-50g pork, beef, or other liver - per person, cut in bite-sized pieces
1/2 onion, chopped
2 Roma Tomatoes, chopped
Sea salt, pepper, and oregano
Optional: 1+ clove of garlic, chopped

Warm a pan, and add the bacon fat. When hot, add onions. Let cook a couple minutes. Add garlic if using, then add liver. Season with salt and pepper. Stir frequently to sear the liver.

As soon as the edges and sides have turned brown, but before it is cooked through, add tomatoes, and oregano. Cover, and turn low to simmer until the tomatoes have softened. The liver should not be too mealy when cooked right. Over cooking liver creates a less desirable texture.

Fish:

Salmon, cod, or other fish can be pan-fried, baked, poached, or grilled. I typically stick to the simple cooking methods, pan-frying in xvoo with salt and pepper, and a drizzle of lemon or lime juice. Cod and other mild white fish are good baked with either the *Parsley Pesto*, or *Basil Pesto*, above.

You can also dip the fish in an egg white bath, then a seasoned ground almond or flour and herb blend, and either fry or bake. Coconut flour gives the fish a nice buttery flavor, and can be used by those on gluten-free diets.

Almond, Pecan, or Coconut Crusted Cod or Mild White Fish:

Place about 1/2 cup ground almond or pecan, or coconut flour on a plate. Add 1/4-1/3 tsp. sea salt, pepper, and a pinch of cayenne pepper, or whatever other seasoning you like, such as dried dill, thyme, or parsley.

In a separate bowl, lightly beat 1 egg, 2 egg whites or 1/4 cup liquid egg white. Dip fish into egg, then roll in the seasoned nut or coconut flour mix, and either place on a baking tray lined with parchment paper, or pan-fry in oil &/or butter.

Cook each side until brown, trying not to over cook. Use a fork to test for doneness. The flesh should be more opaque colored, and easily flake when ready.

Pan-Fried Keta Salmon: *Keta, or Atlantic (Chum) Salmon is less fatty, and has a meaty, but milder flavor which I enjoy.*

Place salmon on a plate, and drizzle a little xvoo, then season with sea salt and pepper.

Pan-fry in a non-stick griddle, (or use a stove top grill pan) beginning with the flesh side down. When it has begun to brown, flip it, add a tad of butter and more seasoning, and let it cook until the flesh easily flakes with a fork. Add a squeeze of lime or lemon juice before serving. Enjoy with *Creamy Coleslaw, Pan-Fried Cabbage*, or *Red Onion & Red Bell Pepper Relish*, below.

Variation:

Dust with coconut or other flour. The easiest way is to pat fish dry. Place a little flour into a small, fine mesh strainer, like a tea strainer, and shake to lightly dust the fish. Season with sea salt, white or black pepper, and dill. Pan-fry as above, in butter, xvoo, or coconut oil.

Red Onion & Red Bell Pepper Relish:

Sauté diced red onion, and red bell pepper in olive oil and/or butter, and season with sea salt and pepper. Add a few drops of balsamic vinegar and low-sodium, wheat-free soy sauce, liquid aminos, or sea salt. Cook until tender. Serve on top of the salmon.

Pan-Fried Cabbage:

1 lg. sweet or yellow onion, sliced
1/2 head of cabbage, sliced horizontally into 1/4 inch wedges in the shape of fettuccine noodles
2+ tsp. each xvoo + butter, or coconut oil + butter
1 tsp. turmeric or curry powder
1/4-1/3 tsp. ground fennel
Sea salt & white pepper

Heat a deep pan, and add oil + butter. Add onions, and let cook 2-3 minutes before adding cabbage. Season with sea salt, turmeric or curry powder, and fennel, stirring to evenly coat the cabbage. (Whole seeds can be ground in a designated coffee grinder).

Cover, and let cook on medium-low heat for about 7-10 minutes, until cabbage has softened. Alternatively, add 1/4 cup bone broth before covering with a lid.

Simple Tangy Tuna Salad:

1 can of better quality tuna, packed in water, drained
1 hard-boiled egg
4 black pitted olives
1/4 red or sweet onion, minced or diced
1/2-1 dill pickle, chopped + 1-2 tbsp. pickle juice

Place ingredients in a bowl, chopping up the egg and olives with a fork until everything is well combined. Taste, and adjust the flavor as desired. It will get better as it sits.

Variations:

- Add a little fresh lemon juice.
- Add 1+ tsp. of a grainy or dijon mustard.
- Add 1+ tbsp. xvoo or avocado oil.
- Add 2+ tbsp. *Mayonnaise* (See recipe taken from NeanderThin, by Ray Audette, below)
- Sub tuna with sardines (or mackerel) packed in olive oil or water, or use both.
- Make this with canned salmon that contains the bones for added calcium.
- Add chopped celery or diced bell pepper.
- Add fresh herbs like chopped parsley, chives, or dill.
- Sub the dill pickle for 1 tbsp. sweet pickle relish.

Serve the *Tangy Tuna Salad* with any of the following *Cucumber Salad* variations.

Cucumber Salad:

1 cucumber, peeled, quartered & chopped
1 fresh tomato, chopped
1/4 red or sweet onion, finely chopped
Juice of 1/4-1/2 lemon
1 tsp. *Carlson Labs Lemon Cod Liver Oil* per person/serving
.5-1 tbsp. xvoo per person
Sea salt & pepper

Combine ingredients in a bowl, and toss gently. Serve with the *Tangy Tuna Salad,* allowing the Tuna (made without oil) to soak up the lemon flavored dressing. Fresh and delicious!

Variations:
•Add chopped sheep, goat, or cow feta cheese
•Add 1/2-1 avocado.
•Add soaked and rinsed wakame seaweed, or dulse.

Dulse is a red seaweed, and one of my favorites. It can be crisped up, somewhat like a bacon substitute. Heat dulse on a tray in the oven set at 175-200° for 5-6 minutes, until it crisps up. Pay attention ~ it burns quickly!

Pressed Red Cabbage Salad:

1/2+ head of red cabbage
1/4 red onion, or 3 scallions, thinly sliced
Any other vibrant colored veggies desired, such as shredded beet, carrot, or diced red pepper
Sea salt & cracked black or white pepper
Fresh citrus (orange, lime, or lemon) *or*
Vinegar of choice (ume plum vinegar is good,

just use a little less salt), apple cider vinegar, or a red or white balsamic vinegar
Oil of choice: xvoo, pecan oil, hazelnut oil, and/or toasted sesame oil
Pinch or two of stevia, or 1-2 tsp. maple syrup
Fresh herbs (parsley, mint, basil, etc.)

Place cabbage and other vegetables in a bowl. Add some sea salt, and either the fresh squeezed citrus (about 1/2 a lemon or lime, 1/4-1/2 a small orange), or a sprinkle of vinegar.

Place some of the oil on your fingers, and squeeze, squeeze, squeeze. The cabbage will begin to darken in color, and shrink in volume.

Add 1+ tbsp. oil of choice, and sprinkle on a pinch or two of stevia, or add the syrup. Toss, and taste. Adjust with more sour flavor, oil, salt, or sweetener as desired. Season with black pepper or other fresh herbs like parsley or mint for a really fresh taste.

If you prefer a coleslaw with mayonnaise, here is the recipe for home made mayonnaise from NeanderThin:

Mayonnaise:

1 egg + 1 egg yolk
1/2 tsp. dry mustard
1/4 tsp. crushed/ fresh ground sea salt
1/4 tsp. white pepper
2 tbsp. lemon juice (about 1 lemon)
1.5 cups light (single origin) olive oil &/or
pecan, hazelnut, or avocado oil

Crack egg + yolk into food processor. Add remaining ingredients except oil. Cover and process 3-5 seconds. With motor running, slowly add oil, and process just until thick and creamy. It should keep for 7 days, or maybe more in a tightly covered jar in the fridge.

Variation: According to the recipe, if using a blender instead of a food processor, skip the extra egg yolk, and use .5 tbsp. less of lemon juice, and .5 cup less of oil.

Creamy Coleslaw:

1/2-1 head green and/or red cabbage
1 carrot, shredded

1/4 red onion, chopped, or 2-3 scallions, sliced

1/2-1 cup *Mayonnaise*, above

Pinch or two of stevia or 1/2-1 tsp. Xylitol or Swerve

Mix all ingredients in a bowl. Adjust seasoning to taste, adding a little more sea salt, or sweetener as desired.

Variations:
• Add chopped pecans (try roasting first for about 10-15 minutes on a parchment-lined baking tray at 300°).
• Add fresh dill.
• Add chopped celery, shredded beat, or diced orange bell pepper.

More simple meal or snack ideas

• 150g(+/-) sliced smoked turkey drumstick with veggie sticks, 1 oz. goat or feta cheese, and 1/2 orange or some cherries.

• 100-150g sliced pre-cooked ham (Carvers, a Canadian brand is lower in sodium) with a few leaves of romaine lettuce, sliced tomato, a few radishes, and a little optional

Mayonnaise, sweet relish, or dijon mustard along with 1 oz. grass-fed or raw cheese, or fresh fruit.

- Fry sliced ham in a pan with a little bacon fat. Flip, top with whole-fat mozzarella, cooking until melted. Top with spicy mustard, and optional chopped arugula.

   Note: *If keeping a store-bought ham around, look for those labeled "lean" or "extra-lean." To minimize sodium, slice, and leave in a pyrex dish in the fridge, covered in water.*

- 2 hard boiled eggs, a piece of crisp cooked, uncured/better quality bacon, romaine lettuce leaves, sliced tomato.

- Chicken or turkey breast meat, or hard boiled eggs prepared like the *Tangy Tuna Salad*, or any of the variations.

- **Deviled Eggs***:* Cut hard boiled eggs in half lengthwise. Scoop out yolk, and mix with regular or spicy dijon mustard, and *Mayonnaise* (recipe above) ~ adding a little at a time to keep mixture somewhat thick and stiff. Season with sea salt and pepper. Spoon mix back into the eggs, and sprinkle fine diced red onion, and paprika on top. These pack well and are delicious!

- Any sort of antipasti with marinated feta cheese, peppers, olives, etc., with some better quality sliced roast beef, salami, or other meats; raw or fermented vegetables, and a little optional fresh fruit.

- 1/2-1 cup 4% fat cottage cheese, plain, or with 1/2 chopped pear, peach, fresh berries or 20-25g of raisins, 1/4 tsp. of cinnamon, and a pinch of stevia; or have with chopped vegetables like celery, radishes, or scallions, or optional chopped roasted hazelnuts &/or pecans.

- A recent favorite snack has been combining 1/2 cup of ricotta cheese with 3/4-1 cup of plain, whole-fat yogurt. During colder months, I let it come up to room temperature before eating. Heating plain ricotta cheese in a heat-proof bowl on a low heat makes a delicious dessert topped with cinnamon.

- 1 cup of whole-fat plain yogurt with optional 1/2-1 scoop of vanilla protein powder stirred in, or a few drops of real vanilla, and a pinch of stevia, or as a treat for those who tolerate, add 1 tsp. raw honey.

- 15 or so cherries and 1 oz. of almonds, pecans, or hazelnuts.

- Fresh, good quality shrimp when available made like a shrimp cocktail with some celery or *Cucumber Salad.*

- Part of an Epic bar or Tanka bar, or some beef, buffalo, turkey, or salmon jerky with some cheese and/or vegetables, or with some pecans and cherries or berries.

- Pair a saltier meat with a juicy fruit, such as sliced ham or prosciutto, or smoked salmon with a sweet seasonal cantaloupe and some juicy cucumber.

- Chilled Gazpacho Soup with chopped avocado, and some fresh or canned Ahi or tuna salad.

- Sardines, eaten from the can, or served on a salad; or quickly pan-fry seasoned sardines or mackerel in olive oil and serve on salad greens with *Vinaigrette Dressing,* above.

- Make a Lettuce Wrap with sliced meat, avocado and/or sliced cheese, tomato, onion, and a little mustard or sliced pickle.

- Have a bowl of bone broth with one of your meals, or make a hearty *Chicken Vegetable Soup* ~ recipes on the website.

- Place sliced roast beef into a bowl, and top with a little bone broth, and sauerkraut.

- Simmer sausages or bratwursts in some bone broth with chopped cabbage, onion, ground fennel, and dried thyme, along with optional chopped tomatoes.

•Alternatively, do as a friend and resident expert on cooking brats does, and simmer them in beer first, along with sliced onions, a few whole fennel seeds, and 1-2 cloves garlic. Enjoy as is, or take them out of the broth to grill, or pan-fry until nicely browned before serving. Serve with the *Pan-Fried Cabbage*, above, and fresh radishes. Top with a big teaspoon of grainy mustard.

•Serve *Pressed Cabbage Salad*, above, with fresh or canned better quality tuna, salmon, mackerel or taco style ground beef or ground turkey.

•Try the *Protein-Rich Eggnog*, or Don's *Chocolate Almond Protein Bar*, below.

Don's Chocolate Almond Protein Bars:

1 cup hemp protein powder
1/4 cup raw almond butter
2-3 oz. water
2-4 pieces of Bakers Brand baking chocolate
4 tsp. Xylitol(Swerve or Xyla brands)

Combine hemp and almond butter in a bowl. Add water to a small pot, then add the chocolate and Xylitol. Gently warm, stirring as needed, until the chocolate is melted, and the Xylitol has dissolved. Add to the hemp mixture. When well combined, form into 'bars' in your hands.

Place on a wax or parchment paper lined tray, and freeze. Keep wrapped and frozen until ready to eat, letting them warm up briefly before eating. Makes 8 bars.

Homemade Yogurt: *Making yogurt is much more cost effective, simple, and delicious!*

2-3 quarts whole milk
1/4 cup of already made yogurt per quart of milk, left at room temp to warm up

Place milk in a pot, and cook on medium heat until it reaches 165° for 30 seconds. Turn off heat, and let the temperature come down to just under 120°. This will help destroy unwanted bacteria. Add about a cup of the milk to the yogurt, stir, then return mixture to the pot. Stir until combined. Pour into jars, then let incubate for around 8 hours, or overnight. We use a Coleman cooler, and wrap a heating pad around the jars, then set to medium. You can watch Don preparing a batch on my Tracy A. Minton-Matesz YouTube channel.

9 BEVERAGES

Coffee or tea can be enjoyed black, or with added butter and/or half and half, or heavy cream. Also good brewed with cinnamon.

If avoiding coffee, *Chicory Coffee,* made with Prewetts Instant Organic Chicory is an excellent tasting, caffeine-free alternative. Follow the link to order the brand we use.

Chicory Coffee: *This makes a great dessert!*

2 tsp. Prewetts Instant Organic Chicory
6 oz. boiling water
2-3 tbsp. heavy cream (as is, or whipped)
1 tsp. Xyla, optional

Place chicory in a mug. Add boiling water, stir, then add cream and Xyla. Stir. Top with a dusting of cinnamon or cocoa as desired.

To order Prewetts: https://www.amazon.com/gp/product/B009ZS9LE4?ie=UTF8

Roasted Dandelion & Roasted Chicory:

Purchase roasted dandelion and roasted chicory separately in bulk. Heat about 1/8 cup of each in a glass or ceramic pot with about 4 cups purified water. Bring just barely up to a boil, then turn it lower, and let it simmer, covered for about 10 minutes.

You can also add a little citrus peel, licorice root, a cinnamon stick, whole cloves, 3-4 cardamon pods, or other chai spices if you like. Drink like coffee, with cream, and a little stevia or natural sweetener as desired.

There are many other healthy coffee alternatives you can check out on my website.

Rose Hips, Hibiscus & Chrysanthemum Tea:

4 cups of purified water
2 tbsp. rose hips, 1 tbsp. hibiscus, and 1 tbsp. of chrysanthemum

These amounts can vary, but I use the most of the rose hips. Place ingredients in a glass or ceramic pot. Simmer on lower heat for about

10-15 minutes. Strain into a glass jar, pressing the herbs to extract all the tea.

You can make a second pressing, by adding a little more water and a pinch more herbs.

Sweeten with a little stevia or Xyla natural sweetener while still warm, then keep chilled. This is a great summer time tea, as it is very cooling and refreshing. Enjoy as is, or mixed half and half with a berry flavored sparkling water, or even with a little cream. It has a lot of potassium and other minerals as well.

Drink purified water, fresh made herbal teas, green, white, red or black teas (which, along with cinnamon, contains manganese, an important mineral that is required in small amounts in the diet), or naturally flavored sparkling or mineral waters.

Avoid sodas or other beverages with corn syrup, artificial flavorings and coloring, and refined sugars.

10 FINAL THOUGHTS

I hope you find these very simple recipes satisfying, and easy to prepare for daily consumption. There are many online sources for more low-carbohydrate recipes. I highly recommend keeping things very simple. There are people who are totally happy to spend time cooking a delicious meal, and there are those who literally do not know how to use a real oven.

If you want to be healthy, you simply must learn how to prepare some basic, simple meals. A diet centered around pre-made, processed foods, fast foods, or restaurant foods will not provide you with the right nourishment you need to recover and maintain good health.

Once upon a time, the matriarch of the household prepared meals for the entire family. She was the real doctor of the household as her lovingly prepared meals, made with natural wholesome, seasonal ingredients helped nourish the minds and bodies of the entire family. In traditional Chinese food therapy, special dishes, using herbs and specific ingredients were prepared for any family member that needed extra help to restore balance.

I have removed my previous macrobiotic books and cookbooks from print as I place a high value on honesty, integrity, and being transparent, and did not feel good about having conflicting information circulating. However, while I no longer advocate an entirely plant-based, or grain-based, vegan diet, my desire was and remains to inspire a return to the kitchen as a means of healing our society, one person at a time.

I hope to bring back the recognition of the sacredness of the role of the nurturer, cook and care taker of the household, which traditionally was the female role. This *is* our most important role or 'profession' ~ to care for and help grow young children into healthy, productive humans.

Whether you are male or female, and live alone or have a family to care for, preparing a nutritious meal is an act of self-love. Every bite you take is either contributing to or taking away from your health ~ physically and mentally.

It is only in recent times that we have been able to purchase any type of 'food' that was first formulated in a lab, then produced in a factory, packaged, shipped, and sold whereby it could be purchased, brought home and be ready in no time by zapping it in a micro-wave. To quote Joel Salatin, "Folks, this ain't normal." Even if it is becoming the new 'norm' it ain't natural, and it ain't healthy.

When choosing what to eat for your meals and/or snacks throughout the day, take a little time to plan. Make some homemade mayonnaise, then make a big batch of *Creamy Coleslaw*, and boil eggs to make *Deviled Eggs*. Make a *Slow Roasted Roast Beef* that you can enjoy for two to three days. While using the oven, roast some chicken drumsticks or turkey thighs or breast at the same time. This will provide you with super easy meals for much of your work week.

Here are a few other tips or considerations for succeeding with *The Trust Your True Nature Diet Low-Carb Plan*:

1. There are many books, bloggers, and doctors promoting plant-based diets. They sound convincing. It has become common place to vilify red meat, while singing the virtues of plants. When people recount their typical meals, they sheepishly ~ as if riddled with guilt ~ interject that they only eat red meat on occasion. Eat red meat, it's very healthy. Eat pork, lamb, wild game, fish, or poultry ~ according to your natural desires, and what is more prominently found in your local, natural environment.

2. Natural fats from animal sources are not the underlying cause of heart disease. Eat healthy, traditional animal fats, especially those intrinsic to the animal flesh foods. Butter, tallow, duck fat, or a good quality lard from pastured animals are preferred sources of fats. Extracted, liquid oils are a much more modern food.

I know most early Europeans never consumed coconuts or coconut oils, or avocado oil for that matter, and had good health. Coconut oil is touted as a super food, but let's be real here. It's an oil, processed from a plant, that comes from a tropical environment. It has its place, but let's keep it on a shelf, and off the pedestal.

3. Many people believe meat, especially red meat to be the cause of their constipation. I used to believe this as well.

We are all under a spell of indoctrination that tells us that we must eat lots of high-fiber foods, and fruits and vegetables, to maintain health, especially of our digestive system. In actuality, most people have never tried eating a mostly animal-based diet, just as our ancestors did for thousands of years, free of our current rates of degeneration and dis-ease. There is reason to believe that it is the *plant* foods that are the greater source of many people's digestive woes and health issues.

Our intestines, digestion, and nutrient requirements resemble those of carnivores, not those of herbivores. For example, natural herbivores have guts that digest fiber, but like other carnivores, we do not. Sure, if you eat enough fiber, and drink enough water, the undigested contents of your colon – fiber – will eventually get pushed out. But this is not natural, and actually causes your intestinal muscles, and the action of peristalsis to weaken.

I had off and on constipation for much of my life. I thought a plant-based diet would resolve that. I ended up with more of a spastic colon, having a huge elimination after I consumed enough fibrous plant foods, and chugged down enough water, which also caused my lower belly to pouch out. Then I would have many days of little elimination, difficult elimination, or a plopping out of contents, followed again after some time by one big show-stopper.

You may not have show-stopper number 2s ~ nor are they necessary ~ while eating a very low-carb diet. You may not eliminate every single day. But neither will you have the downward pressing feeling like you should be having a bowel movement, but can't. Your gut needs time to heal. The muscles need time to regain their ability to work again. Give it time. Just make sure you eat adequate amounts of fat, and take magnesium, as described previously. I also highly suggest investing in a Squatty Potty.

4. If on a budget, perhaps splurge on grass-fed butter, or pastured eggs. Both are higher in vitamin A and Conjugated Linoleic Acid (CLA) which have been studied and found beneficial for helping decrease human breast cancer cell growth, and helping reduce body fat.[8] [9]

A good quality egg will be a deeper hue, nearly orange or even red in color. The yolk will maintain its shape and have a greater height and mass when cracked, versus spreading out, as many commercial eggs will do.

Grass-fed butter will likewise be more yellow. In fact, the fat of grass-fed animals will be more yellowish, less white in color.

---

[8] Conjugated Linoleic Acid Decreases MCF-7 Human Breast Cancer Cell Growth and Insulin-Like Growth Factor-1 Receptor Levels, Springer Link, Amuru and Field, 2009 https://link.springer.com/article/10.1007%2Fs11745-009-3288-4

[9] Conjugated LInoleic Acid Reduces Body Fat Mass in Overweight and Obese Humans, The Journal of Nutrition, Blanksons, Stakkestad, et al., 2000 http://jn.nutrition.org/content/130/12/2943.full

5. **Avoid** commercial plant oils and anything hydrogenated or partially hydrogenated.

6. Plan out your snacks and meals. Don't just start eating handful after handful of nuts, which while they can be healthy in moderate amounts, they should not be in place of a meal.

   If you are trying to lose weight, plan each meal or snack around a healthy protein source. A glass of warmed milk, or a hot morning beverage with some cream can be a stand in 'first meal' but make sure to include a healthy source of protein with whatever is your next meal. It's too easy to grab anything in sight when you wait too long past your first cues of hunger. Don't do it. Especially if you have any issues with blood sugar imbalance, insulin resistance, or sensitivity to carbohydrates.

7. Enjoy non-starchy, crunchy vegetables and greens as desired, yet don't feel obligated to eating them *"because they are supposed to be good for you."* Trust your own cues!

8. Starchy vegetables, like sweet or regular potatoes can also be enjoyed, however, we highly suggest being mindful to keep total quantity of carbohydrates consumed to 100-150g per day or less. I personally believe many people will do best with 75-100g *max*.

9. For the best results with weight loss, and determining which foods you best tolerate, try eliminating *all* grains, beans, breads, and flour products, while minimizing sweeter fruits and starchy vegetables for *at least* one to two months to see how you feel. Make adjustments as needed.

10. I no longer believe 'grains, greens, and beans' to be the pinnacle of health as I had for nearly my entire life. I know I'm taking on a sacred cow here, however people can consume an excess of calories, and still be malnourished. When you eat too few of the most nutrient-dense animal foods *and* fats, and too many processed foods, *and* plant foods that contain less bio-available nutrition ~ in addition to containing naturally occurring toxic substances that can inhibit absorption of essential minerals

~ your system becomes more and more deplete over time. This leads to premature aging and weakening bones as well.

It took me a bit to unwind from these long-standing, mass conscious belief systems, but I have learned to trust *my* true nature, and not get hooked. I witnessed my own accelerated aging and degeneration while eating an entirely plant-based diet, believing I was eating all of nature's most healthful, nutrient-dense foods, however, I was wrong. Our ancestors survived for thousands of years, and a few ice ages eating primarily animal foods. I now prefer to approximate the diet of my own great ancestors rather than pay attention to those who don't have my best interests at heart.

11. Considering the amount of people dealing with digestive issues, irritable bowel syndrome (IBS), allergies, and skin conditions, I hypothesize that many are still in the dark about the potential destruction these so-called healthy vegetables, greens, grains, beans, and other carbohydrate-rich foods can cause to our

gut health, and immune system.

As suggested earlier, keep a food journal (look for my *7-Day Food Mood Journal* on my website), and try eliminating the foods that you are most 'addicted to' eating from those FODMAP and high histamine food lists, linked above.

12. In order to become more 'fat adapted' you will want to keep total carbohydrate consumption to 50g/day or less. It's really not that difficult. Eat as much protein, fat, and non-starchy vegetables as you crave. The more you simplify your diet, at least initially, the easier it will be for you to determine which foods you tolerate well, and which foods you do not. After a few months of greatly simplifying your diet, you may find you no longer crave foods you once thought you couldn't live without!

13. Scientific evidence supporting a low-carbohydrate diet for health does exist, but it goes against the current narrative. There is a seeming agenda to push a more plant-based diet. Do your own research. Trust

your own inner judgement. Experiment. The food debate is heavily influenced by politics and economics. Read research studies carefully. See how the study was set up, who sponsored it, and the outcome. The study conclusions may not add up to what was presented. Most science these days is agenda-based and biased.

14. If you try a really low-carbohydrate diet to begin with, like we did, you may have momentary bouts of nausea, headaches, tiredness, or other malaise. This may indicate that you are not getting adequate sodium. Make sure to get enough good quality sea salt in your diet, and perhaps take a multi-mineral supplement. Hang in there. This will pass!

15. If you experience cramping, make sure to drink plenty of water, eat enough good quality sea salt, and possibly take potassium. We found that adding 1/4 - 1/2 tsp. each of sodium, powdered potassium and magnesium to our drinking water initially helped.

16. Not everyone has a daily elimination. Constipation is when you feel like you really need to defecate, but are having difficulty. The stools are too bulky, or dry, and require a lot of effort. Take 1-3 200-300 mg tablets of magnesium throughout the day with meals, as previously recommended. If the stools become too loose and sticky, cut back your dose. It may take time for your intestines to heal after years of high-fiber, plant-based diets. Alternatively, you can try taking 1 teaspoon of Swedish Bitters prior to your larger meals to help with fat digestion.

17. Organ meats are very nutritious. Liver is among the most nutritious foods. If the thought of eating liver doesn't rock your world, consider taking the Universal Uni Liver Tablets. We each chew 4 of these per day, most days, as shown in the beginning of the meals and recipes section. They are also a good source of calcium.

18. Most importantly, *have patience.* Learn to trust yourself! Make vibrant health your primary goal. Everyone has fluctuating

energy, and minor issues or subtle aches or pains at various times. Don't expect miracles from your diet.

Aim to realize your health goals by:

- Envision yourself as having *already* achieved your desired outcomes, or as I like to say, "keep your eyes on the prize!"

- Find a nice sweet spot whereby you really enjoy your daily meals. Your meals should satisfy your appetite, and be simple enough to prepare so you will actually sustain this way of eating for life.

- Do what you need to do. Trust your inner guidance. Train and move your body. Snap out of self-deceptive brain fogs. Don't let yourself drift into denial. Be real with yourself. Own your responsibilities. Be accountable to your actions. Maintain a decent, clean living environment. Be true to your word, ***and learn to trust yourself***!

11 RESOURCES

www.TrustYourTrueNature.com ~ also at
www.StrongSpiritWoman.com
www.LivingYourTrueNature.blogspot.com -
www.DonMatesz.com
www.DonMatesz.blogspot.com

DietDoctor.com. Once you become a member, you will have access to several great documentaries you can watch, including *Fat Chance, Cereal Killers, parts 1 & 2*, *The Fat Fix*, and more. These documentaries will help you assuage any guilt or doubt over eating a higher fat, low-carbohydrate diet! You can also take his low-carbohydrate challenge, and look for recipes among his fairly extensive database.

Dr. Shawn Baker: Carnivore Diet (Zero Carb Diet Plan) Results and Benefits on YouTube. https://www.youtube.com/watch?v=Gt3tfLVF7Y0v=Gt3tfLVF7Y0

Dr. Ted Naiman, BurnFatNotSugar.com

Books:

The 7-Day Food Mood Journal, Tracy A. Matesz, available Spring, 2018.

Primal Fasting, Don Matesz, now available.

Life Without Bread, How A Low-Carbohydrate Diet Can Save Your Life, Christian B. Allan, Ph.D., and Wolfgang Lutz, M.D.

NeanderThin, Ray Audette with Troy Gilchrist

Good Calories, Bad Calories, Gary Taubes

Fiber Menace: The Truth About the Leading Role of Fiber in Diet Failure, Constipation, Hemorrhoids, Irritable Bowel Syndrome, Ulcerative Colitis, Crohn's Disease and Colon Cancer, Konstantin Monastyrsky

Grain Brain: The Surprising Truth about Wheat, Carbs, and Sugar - Your Brain's Silent Killers, David Perlmutter

Folks, This Ain't Normal, A Farmer's Advice for Happier Hens, Healthier People, and a Better World, Joel Salatin

"Have you tried reading the labels on industrial supermarket food lately? You have to be a chemist and love multisyllabic science-speak to even decipher the labels. Folks, this ain't normal."

"...To return to Prince Charle's point, a culture is identified by its architecture, religion, and food. What differentiates groups of people primarily is not skin color, but how they live, how they think, and how they eat. These are the defining characteristics of any culture...."

~ Joel Salatin, Folks This Ain't Normal, A Farmer's Advice for Happier Hens, Healthier People, and a Better World.

87003926R00083

Made in the USA
Lexington, KY
18 April 2018